A Guide to Chinese
Medicine on the Internet

A Guide to Chinese Medicine on the Internet

Ka wai Fan, PhD

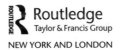

Routledge
Taylor & Francis Group

NEW YORK AND LONDON

First published 2008
by Routledge
270 Madison Ave, New York, NY 10016

Simultaneously published in the UK
by Routledge
2 Park Square, Milton Park, Abingdon, Oxon OX14 4RN

Routledge is an imprint of the Taylor & Francis Group, an informa business

© 2008 Taylor & Francis

Printed and bound in the United States of America on acid-free paper by
Edwards Brothers, Inc.

Due to the ever-changing nature of the Internet, Web site names and
addresses, though verified to the best of the publisher's ability, should not
be accepted as accurate without independent verification.

Cover design by Jennifer M. Gaska.

Library of Congress Cataloging in Publication Data
  A guide to Chinese medicine on the Internet / Ka Wai Fan.
     p.; cm.
  Includes bibliographical references.
  1. Medicine, Chinese—Computer network resources—Directories. 2.
Internet addresses—Directories. 3. Web sites—Directories. I. Title.
  [DNLM: 1. Medicine, Chinese Traditional—Resource Guides. 2.
Internet—Resource
  Guides. WB 39 F199g 2007]
  R601.F283 2007
  610.285025—dc22

                                                    2007045395

ISBN10: 0-7890-3199-X (hbk)
ISBN10: 0-7890-3200-7 (pbk)
ISBN10: 0-2038-8932-0 (ebk)

ISBN13: 978-0-7890-3199-0 (hbk)
ISBN13: 978-0-7890-3200-3 (pbk)
ISBN13: 978-0-2038-8932-9 (ebk)

This project has taken nearly two years to compile. I would like to express my heartfelt thanks to Fiona S. N. Lau, Frances Tin, Samuel Gilbert, and Dr. G. A. Plum for their help.

ABOUT THE AUTHOR

Ka wai Fan, PhD, is a full-time lecturer in the Chinese Civilization Center, City University of Hong Kong; an honorary adjunct assistant professor in the School of Chinese Medicine at the Chinese University of Hong Kong; and honorary visiting fellow (2006-2009) at the Center for Traditional Chinese Science and Civilization in The Institute for the History of Natural Science, Chinese Academy of Sciences, Beijing. He received his PhD, MPhil, and BA all from the Department of History, Chinese University of Hong Kong. He worked as an assistant professor in the Institute of History, National Tsinghua University, Taiwan. His research interests include the history of Chinese medicine and online information on Chinese medicine. He has written several publications on both the online resources of Chinese medicine, and the history of Chinese medicine.

CONTENTS

Introduction

Over the past few decades, Chinese medicine, being a kind of complementary and alternative medicine (CAM), has become a growing focus all over the world. This is because Traditional Chinese Medicine (TCM) has been playing an important role in the prevention and cure of diseases and the prolongation of life, through methods such as acupuncture, herbal therapies, and Qigong. More and more people are paying attention to Chinese medicine, although the Chinese medical system is a non-Western medical system.[1]

The Internet is being increasingly used in conjunction with research: to share information; to disseminate findings; and to publicize projects and organizations. At the same time, the ability to sift through the ever-increasing amounts of information made available online to find quality and accurate data is becoming more important every day. The Internet is a very important search tool for faculty members and students. Currently, many disciplines are dependent on the Internet for the dissemination of information. In fact, many professors and scholars use online resources to pursue their own research.[2] However, simply using a search engine, such as Google or Yahoo, to look for information will not necessarily lead one to quality resources, and is more likely to provide a large number of unordered results to sift through. Many useless items are also included in the results, and the quality or reliability of the search results cannot be ensured. In a survey of the information available on the World Wide Web (WWW) about the use of herbal medicine in the treatment of cancer, most sites were found to be inadequate in a number of areas, including bias, accuracy, clear presentation of sources of information, and regularity of updates.[3]

A Guide to Chinese Medicine on the Internet

A great deal of Chinese and English-language information about Chinese medicine is available online. However, this information is not reviewed by experts and the authors of such information may not be professionals in the field represented by the information. Many people are concerned that the information about Chinese medicine that is available on the Internet may be wrong, useless, and even harmful if followed without further advice. The purpose of this book is to provide a guide to the information about Chinese medicine that is available on the WWW in order to help interested people find up-to-date and reliable information and learn about new developments in Chinese medicine easily and quickly. It should be noted that the book does not encourage the use of any particular Chinese medical therapy for the treatment of any disease. If readers want to use Chinese medicine for treatment purposes, they should consult their doctor or a qualified professional rather than accept at face value what is stated on a Web site. Any information posted on the Internet should only be used for reference purposes, not for making any treatment decision.

Although there are guides available for CAM online resources,[4] there does not seem to be any publication that functions as a guide to using the Internet to research Chinese medicine.[5] This book provides a categorized listing of Web sites related to Chinese medicine, with a brief description of each site's content. In addition, it discusses guidelines for searching, cataloging, and evaluating Web sites concerned with Chinese medicine based on the author's personal experience as a user.

CHINESE MEDICINE AS COMPLEMENTARY AND ALTERNATIVE MEDICINE (CAM)

In 1998 the United States government established The National Center for Complementary and Alternative Medicine (NCCAM) as one of the twenty-seven institutes and centers that make up the renowned National Institutes of Health (NIH) within the U.S. Department of Health and Human Services. NCCAM is dedicated to exploring complementary and alternative healing practices in the context of rigorous science; to training CAM researchers; and to disseminating authoritative information to the public and to professionals. So what is CAM? As defined by NCCAM, CAM is a group of diverse medical and health care systems, practices, and products that are not presently considered part of conventional medicine. Complementary medicine is used together with conventional medicine. Alternative medicine is used in place of conventional medicine.

What is the meaning of "conventional medicine"? Conventional medicine is medicine as practiced by holders of MD (medical doctor) or DO (doctor of osteopathy) degrees and by allied health professionals, such as physical therapists, psychologists, and registered nurses. Terms for conventional medicine include allopathy; Western, mainstream, orthodox, regular medicine, and biomedicine. Some conventional medical practitioners are also practitioners of CAM.[6] As NCCAM is an authoritative institute, its definition is widely accepted. Many CAM Web sites copy this definition and link it to NCCAM.

Under "Medical Subject Healings" the National Medical Library has an entry headed "Alternative Medicine" (also used in MEDLINE): "An unrelated group of non-orthodox therapeutic practices, often with explanatory systems that do not follow conventional biomedical explanations" (MeSH Term Working Group, NIH, 1993). Between 1963 and 1993, the relevant entry had been headed "Therapeutic Cults" and read "non-orthodox therapeutic systems which have no satisfactory scientific explanation for their effectiveness."[7]

Presently, the description of alternative medicine or complementary medicine (with a definition of "alternative medicine" combined with that of "complementary therapies") under the heading "Medical Subject Healings" in the National Medical Library reads:

> Therapeutic practices which are not currently considered an integral part of conventional allopathic medical practice. They may lack biomedical explanations but as they become better researched some (physical therapy, diet, acupuncture) become widely accepted whereas others (humors, radium therapy) quietly fade away, yet are important historical footnotes. Therapies are termed as complementary when used in addition to conventional treatments and as alternative when used instead of conventional treatment.[8]

The difference between the two descriptions is very apparent. The former bluntly stated that CAM had no satisfactory scientific explanation for the effectiveness of any therapies, whereas the latter—while still stating that CAM may lack biomedical explanations—concedes that some CAM therapies may become widely accepted as they become better researched.

The Alternative Medicine Homepage is maintained by University of Pittsburgh librarian Charles Wessel, who is an authority on CAM Internet resources. He provides three definitions on his Web site. The first definition cites the National Library of Medicine stated previously. The second definition states that "[CAM] as medical interventions [are] not taught at United States medical schools or [are] not available at United States hospitals." This definition comes from David Eisenberg of the Harvard Medical School, who with his colleagues conducted surveys into the use of CAM in the United States between 1993 and 1998. Eisenberg says that "Alternative Medicine can be defined as medical interventions that are neither taught widely in US medical schools nor generally available in US hospitals."[9] This definition first appeared in an article by Eisenberg in 1993 and was repeated in another article in 1998. David Eisenberg's articles are widely cited and his definitions have therefore found their way onto the Web.

The third definition provided on the Alternative Medicine Homepage comes from the Panel on Definition and Description, CAM Research Methodology Conference, Office of Alternative Medicine, National Institutes of Health, Bethesda, Maryland, April 1995:

> Complementary and alternative medicine as a broad domain of healing resources that encompasses all health systems, modalities, and practices and their accompanying theories and beliefs, other than those intrinsic to the politically dominant health system of a particular society or culture in a given historical period. CAM includes all such practices and ideas self-defined by their users as preventing or treating illness or promoting health and well being. Boundaries within CAM and between the CAM domain and the domain of the dominant system are not always sharp or fixed.[10]

This definition does not focus on distinguishing between CAM and conventional medicine; instead, CAM is viewed as a collection of healing resources with its own theories and beliefs.

The *Oxford Concise Medical Dictionary* is written by medical experts, and updated from time to time. The *Oxford Concise Medical Dictionary* (fifth edition, 1998) has the following entry under the heading "alternative medicine":

> The various systems of "healing" including homeopathy, herbal remedies, hypnosis and faith healing, that are not regarded as part of orthodox treatment by the medical profession, especially when offered by unregistered practitioners. Most of the treatments are of unproven benefit but are tried by sufferers of chronic or incurable conditions when orthodox treatment has failed. Many alternative therapies are ridiculed by the medical profession, but acupuncture and osteopathy are now generally accepted to be of value in some circumstances. The extent to which individual registered practitioners indulge in or spurn these therapies varies enormously but is governed by the overriding principle (laid down by the General Medical Council) that shared care is only permitted if the registered practitioner remains in overall control; this is often unacceptable to those practicing alternative medicine.[11]

Alternative medicine is defined as *not* being part of orthodox medicine; the examples of therapies given only serve the point of letting us know what therapies belong under the heading of alternative medicine, without thereby "approving" of them in any way. According to the dictionary, alternative medicine may be said to have the following four major characteristics: (1) It is a healing (or medical) system but not part of orthodox medicine; (2) it is offered by unregistered practitioners, not the medical profession; (3) the treatments of alternative medicine are of unproven benefit; and (4) sufferers use alternative medicine when orthodox treatment has failed. In addition, the dictionary offers no description of "complementary medicine" directing readers to go to a cross-reference "see *alternative* medicine."

In 2002, the *Oxford Concise Medical Dictionary* published its sixth edition. It is interesting that there is now no entry "alternative medicine" it having been replaced by an entry: "complementary medicine," thus only directing us to "see *complementary* medicine," which is described as follows:

> Complementary medicine—various forms of therapy that are viewed as complementary to conventional medicine. These include (but are not confined to) osteopathy, acupuncture, homeopathy, massage, reflexology and reiki. Previously, complementary therapies were regarded as an alternative to conventional therapies, and the two types were considered to be mutually exclusive (hence the former names alternative medicine and fringe medicine). However, many practitioners now have dual training in conventional and complementary therapies. There is very limited provision for complementary medicine within the confines of the National Health Service.[12]

The difference between the two editions is very noticeable, the sixth edition having effectively recast alternative medicine as complementary medicine. No longer being placed in an oppositional position to conventional medicine, complementary medicine is now viewed as complementary to conventional medicine.[13] According to the sixth edition of the dictionary, complementary medicine may be said to have the following three major characteristics: (1) CAM is used as complementary to conventional medicine, to be used when conventional medicine has failed; (2) CAM is offered by many registered practitioners who are trained in both conventional and complementary therapies; (3) The National Health Service in the United Kingdom also provides some (although very limited) complementary therapies for sufferers. The changed definitions in the two editions undoubtedly reflect a growth in the medical profession's understanding of CAM and also observable trends in the provision of CAM.

To sum up, the definitions reflect our changing understanding of CAM. Previously, as the *Oxford Concise Medical Dictionary* (fifth edition) pointed out, many alternative therapies were ridiculed by the medical profession. One of the differences between CAM and conventional medicine is that CAM is considered to be nonscientific. Marcia Angell and Jerome Kassirer say that

> It [CAM] has not been scientifically tested and its advocates largely deny the need for testing. . . . Alternative medicine also distinguishes itself by an ideology that largely ignores biologic mechanisms, often disparages modern medicine science, and relies on what are purported to be ancient practices and natural remedies.[14]

It is difficult for the medical profession to accept CAM when CAM is defined as nonscientific and is not taught in medical schools. However, when searching for CAM information online, the author finds that, first, more and more professional medical journals publish research, case reports, and clinical reports about CAM, and CAM journals also state that published articles are peer-reviewed and based on scientific and biomedical research.

Second, according to a survey, there is tremendous heterogeneity and diversity in content, format, and requirements among courses in complementary and alternative medicine at U.S. medical schools.[15] For example, the Stanford University Faculty of Medicine provides a CAM program on the topic of "Successful Aging."[16]

Third, university libraries, such as those at the University of British Columbia and McMaster University,[17] provide professional CAM information on the Web. Special research centers have also been established, such as the Oregon Center for Complementary and Alternative Medicine in neurological disorders, and the Richard and Hinda Rosenthal Center for Complementary and Alternative Medicine at Columbia University.[18] Many research centers for CAM therapies are funded by NACCM. In other words, CAM is not being totally rejected by the university medical education system.

Chinese medicine, as part of CAM, also shows these trends. Chinese medicine, including acupuncture, Qigong and herbals, continually edges toward the mainstream of conventional medicine, and more serious research is being conducted both scientifically and clinically. Using scientific methods to study Chinese medicine is now mainstream. In some European countries and the United States, there are regulations governing the practice of Chinese medicine, especially acupuncture treatment. Many medical journals publish articles related to Chinese medicine in the English-speaking world. The University of Westminster and the University of Middlesex, both in the United Kingdom, provide degree courses in Chinese medicine, of course using English to teach.

In Chinese people's minds, Chinese medicine is not CAM. Although universities of TCM in China teach Chinese medicine, half of their courses actually teach Western medicine, and research into Chinese medicine in China emphasizes the integration of Chinese and Western medicine. What is Chinese medicine? This question is very difficult to answer. NCCAM offers the following definition of TCM:

> Traditional Chinese Medicine (TCM) is the current name for an ancient system of health care from China. TCM is based on a concept of balanced Qi (pronounced "chee"), or vital energy, that is believed to flow throughout the body. Qi is proposed to regulate a person's spiritual, emotional, mental, and physical balance and to be influenced by the opposing forces of yin (negative energy) and yang (positive energy). Disease is proposed to result from the flow of Qi being disrupted and yin and yang becoming imbalanced. Among the components of TCM are herbal and nutritional therapy, restorative physical exercises, meditation, acupuncture, and remedial massage.[19]

NCCAM's description seems only to emphasize the concept of Qi. Actually, Chinese medicine is based on philosophical systems (the theories of yin-yang, five phases and Qi), the view of the body (zang-fu—internal organs) system, system of Meridians, acupoints), the causes of diseases, diagnosis, treatments, etc. Wikipedia describes the TCM as follows:

> Traditional Chinese Medicine is a range of traditional medical practices used in China that developed during several thousand years. These practices include herbal medicine, acupuncture, and massage. TCM is a form of *Oriental medicine,* which in-

cludes other traditional East Asian medical systems such as Japanese and Korean medicine. TCM says processes of the human body are interrelated and constantly interact with the environment. Therefore the theory looks for the signs of disharmony in the external and internal environment of a person in order to understand, treat and prevent illness and disease. TCM theory is based on a number of philosophical frameworks including the Theory of Yin-yang, the Five Elements, the human body Meridian system, Zang Fu theory, and others. Diagnosis and treatment are conducted with reference to these concepts. TCM does not usually operate within a scientific paradigm but some practitioners make efforts to bring practices into an evidence-based medicine framework.[20]

Wikipedia's description of Chinese medicine is very concise and clear.

HOW TO EVALUATE WEB SITES RELATED TO CHINESE MEDICINE

How does one evaluate the advantages and disadvantages of Web sites? This is a very critical point when searching on the Internet. However, due to each discipline having its own rules and practices, it is very difficult to arrive at general rules that are suitable for all disciplines. Robert Harris's *CARS Checklist* is a general tool that offers some general criteria for evaluating the quality of Web sites. A summary of the *CARS Checklist for Research Source Evaluation* follows:

- Credibility: Trustworthy source, author's credentials, evidence of quality control, known or respected authority, organizational support.
- Accuracy: Up-to-date, factual, detailed, exact, comprehensive, audience and purpose reflect intentions of completeness and accuracy.

- Reasonableness: Fair, balanced, objective, reasoned, no conflict of interest, absence of fallacies or slanted tone.
- Support: Listed sources, contact information, available corroboration, claims supported, documentation supplied.[21]

These are general rules for the evaluation of Web sites. Medical and medicine-related Web sites are likely to make suggestions for treatment or guide readers to adopt / give up some form of treatment. Therefore, the accuracy and reliability of the information provided may well be affected by the author's opinions and have resulted in the information being subjective rather than objective. The author browsed the Web for the topic "how to evaluate medical information on the Internet," and found that the criteria used for evaluation of such information show no great differences.

There are a number of questions any user of the Web interested in medical information should ask: Who is providing the information? Who is paying for the site? Web sites by governments, universities, or other academic institutions, professional associations, and research foundations are among the best sources for scientifically sound health and medical information. What is the purpose of this page? Who is the intended audience? Is the information on this Web site peer-reviewed? Is the information based on scientific evidence and evidence-based medicine? In addition, the reader should be very careful when consulting Web sites that sell pharmaceuticals and provide medical services. It is not easy, and perhaps impossible, for people who are not medical experts to differentiate between Web sites that offer information based on scientific evidence and evidence-based medicine and those whose information is not scientifically based.

Lillian Brazin, in her book *Guide to Complementary and Alternative Medicine on the Internet,* offers one more piece of advice, which is to look out for an official "seal of approval":

> Does it bear the "HONCode" logo? (This code is awarded to sites that meet the HONCode of Conduct). . . . its (Health on the Net Foundation) mission is to guide Internet searchers to reliable and useful online medical and health information. It sets ethical standards for those who develop health and medi-

cal Web sites. . . . URAC (American Accreditation Healthcare Commission) aims to help consumers identify sites that meet high accountability and quality standards. URAC lists the accredited Web sites with the name of the company that produces the sites. The sites are reviewed annually, and the date the accreditation expires is listed. . . . For a good guide to determining a CAM site's credibility or the validity of its claims, check out Quackwatch (http://www.quackwatch.com).[22]

This is a good suggestion, but unfortunately only a few Web sites are evaluated by the Health on the Net Foundation, the American Accreditation Healthcare Commission, or Quackwatch.

Generally speaking, Web sites about Chinese medicine should provide information that is credible and accurate, and the approach taken to information should be a reasonable one. It is just as important that the site's design is user-friendly, i.e., information is easy to find and readable, and the icons are easy to use, etc.

Another issue of the Web site is its accessibility, which requires the host server to be stable and always online. According to the author's experience, Web sites in Mainland China are often disconnected and even missing, and are slow to download Web pages.

As mentioned, Web sites provided by governments, universities, academic institutions, professional associations, research foundations, and nonprofit organizations are among the best sources of scientifically sound health and medical information. The most reliable authors of information available on the Web are professional associations that publish or co-publish academic journals (not newsletters), preferably with reputable publishers.

If readers want to know the effectiveness of the treatment of Chinese medicine, they should consult searchable journal databases, such as Academic Search Premier, ProQuest, ScienceDirect, Springerlink, ISI Thomas, Elsevier Wiley Science, etc. Much information can be found on these databases. You may say that, "I do not pay for a subscription, so I will not be able to see the full text" or "I am not a doctor, so what are the advantages of browsing these databases?" As most of the journals in these databases are peer-reviewed, reading the abstract of an article is a good way to start—especially since abstracts are both published in full and freely available. Generally speaking, abstracts of medical articles include purposes, methods, and results.

A Web site may also provide good suggestions for further searching information on Chinese medicine. As the Web site of California Medial Association points out, take advantage of Internet reviews and annotated links to other internet resources. For some health and medical topics, there are an overwhelming number of possible sources of information. How can you tell which of the many sources are worth exploring? Good starting points are sites that collect links to resources by topic, and particularly useful are those that also review sites, using expertise from experts, practitioners, and/or librarians. Some examples of such collected and reviewed lists are Medical Matrix, HealthWeb, Health and Medical Informatics Digest, MedWeb, and some of the sites of professional medical organizations as well as university or research sites. Published guides, like the many Internet books now in print, may provide useful pointers but can be out-of-date quickly due to the volatile nature of the Internet.[23]

Readers should familiarize themselves with two or three reliable Web sites about Chinese medicine, sites you can trust or that have been reviewed or at least mentioned favorably in books or by experts. If you find a new Web site that seems to contradict much of what is found on a site that is familiar to you, you should be very careful.

NCCAM reminds you of what you should know and avoid. The NCCAM Web site identifies the medical circumstances under which complementary and alternative therapies are appropriate; explains how to find out what scientific studies have been done on the safety and effectiveness of specific treatments; and offers guidelines about evaluating statements made about the effectiveness of a given therapy.

THE BASIC TERMS OF CHINESE MEDICINE

After browsing many Web sites about Chinese medicine, readers will have come across a variety of basic concepts, terms, and theories of Chinese medicine. In order to assist readers in browsing the

Web sites listed in this book, the author has selected thirty-six terms and provided very brief descriptions (according to the authoritative references). The author also recommends Chen Hua's book *Zhong yi de ke xue yuan li* (*Outline of Sinomedicine,* available at: http://healther .stormloader.com),[24] as it offers descriptions of Chinese medical terms and theories. It may be seen as an introduction to Chinese medicine.

acupressure: A method of treatment involving the application of finger pressure at acupuncture points.[25]

acupuncture: The practice of puncturing the body with metal needles (steel, gold, or silver) at specific points in order to regulate construction, defense, Qi, and the blood.[26]

acupuncture point (or acupoint; also xue wei, xue dao): A place on the surface of the body where Qi and blood of the channels and network vessels gather or pass. Through the channels and network vessels, points are connected to other parts of the body and notably the bowels and viscera, whose state of health they can reflect. Various stimuli such as needling, moxibustion, massage, acupressure, and electroacupuncture can be applied at points to regulate internal functions.[27]

Bencao Gang Mu (also Compendium of *Materia Medica*): Bencao Gang Mu, a dictionary of Chinese herbs, was written by Li Shi Zhen (1518-1593). It consists of fifty-two volumes, with more than 1.9 million characters, and more than 1,100 pictures. The book lists 1,892 "medical materials" comprising herbs, animals, and minerals with 11,096 formulae being used in the past.[28]

CAM: Complementary and alternative medicine.

channels or meridians (also jing mai, jing luo): They are the passages through which Qi and blood circulate, correlate the viscera with the limbs, connect the upper and lower parts with the interior and exterior of the body, and regulate the mechanisms of the various parts of the body. These include the Jing-mai (the channels) and Luo-mai (the collateral channels), and hence, make the human body an organic whole.[29] A distinction is made between regular channels, usually referred to as the twelve channels, and extraordinary vessels. The twelve channels, together with Renmai (the anterior midline channel) and Dumai (the posterior midline channel), are called the fourteen channels.

cupping: A method of treatment involving the application of suction to skin to draw out blood and sometimes pus. Cupping is also called "fire cupping" because the suction is produced when, for example, a lighted alcohol swab placed inside the cup burns the oxygen to create a vacuum after the cup has been placed on the skin.[30]

dietetic therapy (also dietary therapy, Shi liao): It refers to the cure method of using the different nature and nutrients of the food to regulate Qi, blood, and yin and yang of zangfu organs.[31]

eight principles: Identification of disease patterns by eight fundamental principles, namely interior and exterior, cold and heat, vacuity and repletion, and yin and yang.[32]

electroacupuncture: A method of acupuncture in which an electrical current is applied to needles inserted in the body in order to produce a combined needle and electrical stimulus.[33]

five flavors (also Wu wei): Acridity, sourness, sweetness, bitterness, and saltiness. Medicinals or foodstuffs of different flavors with different actions.[34]

five phases (also five elements or Wu xing): The ancients thought that the five kinds of materials—metal, wood, water, fire, and earth—were the indispensable and most fundamental elements in constituting the universe. These were bound by enhancing, inhibiting and restraining relationships between them. They were also in constant motion and change. In Traditional Chinese Medicine, they are used to explain and expand on a series of medical problems by comparing and deducing from such properties and mutual relationships.[35] Each of the five viscera is associated with one of the five phases: Liver-wood, Heart-fire, Spleen-earth, Lung-metal, Kidney-water.

four examinations (or four diagnoses): The four examinations, inspection (or looking), listening and smelling, inquiry (or asking), and palpation, provide the raw data for diagnosis.[36]

four qi (also four natures): The four natures of medicinals: cold, heat, warmth, and coolness. Cold medicinals are those effective in treating heat patterns, whereas hot medicinals are those effective in treating cold patterns. Warm and cool medicinals are medicinals with mild hot or cold natures. In addition, there is also a balanced nature whose nature is neither predominantly hot nor cold.[37]

herbalism (also Bencao, herbal medicine): The medical use of preparations that contain exclusively plant material.[38]

Huangdi neijing: The *Huangdi Neijing* (Yellow Emperor's Inner Classic) is likely the most seminal medical text of ancient China. The theoretical foundations of Chinese medicine are systematically covered. The work is comprised of two texts, each of eighty-one chapters or treatises in a question and answer format between the mythical Yellow Emperor (Huangdi) and His ministers. The first text, *Su wen* (Plain Questions) covers the theoretical foundation of Chinese medicine, diagnostic methods and treatment methods. The second and generally less cited text, *Ling shu* (Spiritual Pivot), deals with acupuncture in great detail. [39]

Ji xing: Medicinal preparation. The final form in which medicinals (usually the various ingredients of a formula) are administered, taken, or applied. Commonly used preparations are decoction, pill, powder, wine, and paste.[40]

Jin gui yao lue fang lun (also Jin gui yao lue, Synopsis of Prescriptions of the Golden Chamber): A medical book of three volumes by Zhang Ji (Zhang Zhongjing) of the Eastern Han

Dynasty, completed before 206, it contains twenty-five chapters. The first chapter is a general treatise on the consequences of diseases in the order of organs and meridians; Chapters 2 to 17 deal with the symptoms and treatment of some forty internal diseases; Chapters 18 to 19 with the symptoms and treatment of external disease and dermopathies; Chapters 20 to 22 with gynecopathies and obstetric problems. The other three chapters contain some other prescriptions and prohibited diets. It is the first systematic monograph in China on internal diseases, not only summarizes medical experiences before the Han Dynasty, but also offers the treatment of disease on the basis of differentiation of symptoms and signs and general principles for the formulation of prescriptions. The 262 prescriptions it contains are very valuable clinically even today. [41]

Kampo medicine: The form of Chinese medicine practiced in Japan.[42]

meditation: Meditation is a state of mind which does not seek to manipulate thoughts and emotions but merely to allow them to settle.[43]

moxibustion: A method of applying a heating stimulus to the body by burning the dried and sifted leaf particles from the herb mugwort on or close to the skin, with the aim of freeing Qi and blood, coursing Qi, dispersing cold, eliminating dampness and warming yang. Moxibustion is divided into two distinct methods: indirect moxibustion and direct moxibustion.[44]

Nan jing (also Classic on Medical Problem, Difficult Classic, or Huangdi's Classic on 81 Medical Problem): A medical book completed before the Eastern Han dynasty, attributed to Qin Yueren. Complied in the form of questions and answers, the book mainly deals with the basic theories of TCM, including such aspects as physiology, pathology, anatomy, diagnosis, and treatment. Of eighty-one problems dealt with in the book, problems one to twenty-two are on pulse study. Problems twenty-three to twenty-nine are on the meridians and collaterals. Problems thirty to forty-seven are on the zang-fu organs and the viscera. Problems forty-eight to sixty-one are on diseases. Problems sixty-two to sixty-eight are on acupoints, and problems sixty-nine to eighty-one are on acupuncture.[45]

Oriental medicine: Oriental medicine includes Chinese medicine, Japanese Medicine (Kampo medicine) and Korean Medicine. Japanese Medicine and Korean Medicine are based on TCM, sharing the same medical theories and practices. Sometimes, oriental medicine only means Chinese medicine.

Qi (also Chi, vital energy): Qi refers (1) to the refined materials which are highly nutritious and circulate in the body, analogous to the "Essence principle" or "Virtue principle"; (2) to the functional activities of the viscera and tissues; and (3) to respiratory gases.[46]

Qigong (also Qi-qong, Qi gong): Exercise consisting in controlling respiration and calming the mind and having the ultimate goal of improving physical health, mental alertness, and preventing and treating disease. Nowadays, a broad distinction is made between quiescent Qi cultivation and active Qi cultivation. Quiescent Qi cultivation consists of breathing exercises in lying, sitting, or standing posture aimed at regulating and containing true Qi. Active Qi cultivation consists in gentle rhythmical movements and self-massage.[47]

Shang han lun (also Shang Han Za Bing Lun, On Cold Damage): The world's most famous clinical medical book was written by Zhang Zhongjing around 200 BC. It includes the *Shang Han Lun* and the *Synopsis of Prescriptions of the Golden Chamber*. The *Shang Han Lun* covers diseases due to external attack, also known as "traumatized by coldness." The *Synopsis of Prescriptions of the Golden Chamber* covers all the clinical difficulties and complications of internal damage. The *Shang Han Lun* is the oldest complete clinical textbook in world medical history, and the *Shang Han Lun* and the *Synopsis of Prescriptions of the Golden Chamber* are two of the four most important medical classics which students must study in Chinese medical education.[48]

Shennong bencao jing (Shennong's herbal Classic): An herb book, the earliest herbal work in China, authorship unknown, completed at about the turn of the Qin Dynasty. The original book is long lost, seen only in other herbal literature of later generations. The existing texts are all complied by later editors. The book begins with a general introduction dealing with the theory of *Materia Medica* and the composition of prescriptions. In the following parts, medicinal materials are classified into three classes according to their functions. In addition to such important theories as different roles played by the medicines within a prescription including the monarch, the minister, the assistant, and the guide, the combination of yin and yang, and the seven different effects in compatibility of ingredients, the book also elaborates on the different names, properties, flavor, functions, and indications of each time. As a comprehensive summary of the achievement in the field before the Qin and Han Dynasty, which laid a foundation for the theoretic system of Chinese *Materia Medica,* this book has high historic and scientific value.[49]

seven affects (also seven qing): Joy, anger, anxiety, thought, sorrow, fear, and fright. In excess the seven affects can be a cause of disease. Powerful or lasting emotions and certain mental activities can damage yin, yang, Qi, blood, and eventually the bowels and viscera.[50]

six excesses (also six yin): Excess or untimeliness of the six Qi (wind, cold, summer heat, damp, dryness, and fire) that invade the body through the exterior to cause disease.[51]

Taiji (also Tai Chi, Taiji quan, Taiji chuan): A system of movements and postures rooted in ancient Chinese philosophy and martial arts used to enhance mental and physical health.[52]

Traditional Chinese Medicine (also TCM): Described previously.

traditional medicine: Traditional medicine is the sum total of the knowledge, skills, and practices based on the theories, beliefs, and experiences indigenous to different cultures, whether explicable or not, used in the maintenance of health as well as in the prevention, diagnosis, improvement, or treatment of physical and mental illness.[53]

Tuina (also Tui na, an mo): Chinese massage. Rubbing, pressing, or other manipulation of the body for the treatment and prevention of disease. Massage helps to free the channels and vessels, and also helps to disinhibit the joints. By stimulating the movement of Qi and blood, it can regulate the function of the bowels and viscera, and increase resistance to disease.[54]

Wen Bing (also warm disease): Any of various heat (febrile) diseases characterized by rapid onset and shifts, pronounced heat signs, and a tendency to form dryness and damage yin.[55]

yin-yang: These are general terms for the two opposites of matters and phenomena in nature, which are interrelated and opposed to each other. They represent not only two different matters in opposition but two opposite aspects in the same entity. In Traditional Chinese Medicine, they are used to summarize and explain problems in the fields of anatomy, physiology, pathology, diagnosis, treatment, etc.[56]

Zang fu (also viscera, zangfu): The five viscera are organs of the chest and abdomen: heart, lung, spleen, liver, and kidney. The pericardium is considered a sixth viscus in channel theory. The six bowels (paired by a functional relationship with their respective viscera) are the stomach, small intestine, large intestine, gallbladder, bladder, and triple burner. The function of the viscera is to produce and store essence, while that of the bowels is to decompose food and convey waste.[57]

When searching for information on Chinese medicine, the terms used in Chinese medicine and Western medicine are mixed up. Chinese medicine is traditional but scientifization and modernization are mainstream features in the development of Chinese medicine. Therefore, to use Internet search engines effectively any search should combine Chinese medical terms with Western medical terms, such as "acupuncture and cancer" or "Taiji and diabetes." To express

Chinese medical terms in English, Chinese medical terms should be replaced by their simple English equivalents; examples are meridians and acupoints, which are the standard English terms for Chinese terms. There are also standard codes for the location of meridians and acupoints for non-Chinese speaker. The Chinese traditional medicine and *Materia Medica* subject headings consists of 6,938 subject headings, listed mainly according to the order followed in the Pinyin system. There are fourteen main subject headings and fifty-nine sub-subject headings.[58] If readers can refer to the subject headings listed in the book, time will be saved in running a search on the Internet. All in all, we also need to pay attention to related terms such as complementary and alternative medicine, oriental medicine and traditional medicine, when searching for information on Chinese medicine on the Internet.

This book has collected relevant Web sites mainly in Chinese and English, and some in Japanese. Chinese Web sites are also divided into traditional or simplified Chinese. The former is common in Taiwan and Hong Kong, and the latter in Mainland China and Singapore. When browsing different Chinese databases and Web sites, readers should take care to choose the right code (Big5 for traditional Chinese and GB for simplified Chinese).

CLASSIFICATION OF WEB SITES
ON CHINESE MEDICINE

This book is intended for an English-speaking audience who may not be familiar with Chinese and Japanese Web sites of Chinese medicine. The author considers (1) that the classification offered here should prove useful to librarians when building an electronic library for Chinese studies; and (2) that the list of Web sites should prove useful not only to people interested in issues of health and illness, but also to practitioners and researchers of Chinese medicine and CAM.

In this book, Web sites are grouped into the following chapters: portals and general Web sites, organizations, libraries, schools, journals, databases, and history and philosophy. Readers should be reminded that (1) a number of Web sites listed in this book are linked to each other. If a certain organization also publishes journals, it will be introduced as two entries in separate chapters. (2) Some Chinese and Japanese Web sites that do not have English titles will be translated.

Portals and General Web sites

As a way of introducing the topic, useful portals and general Web sites are listed in this chapter, comprising a multiplicity of Web sites.

Organizations

This chapter will list Web sites maintained by governments and official organizations as well as sites maintained by academic associations and societies. The author considers information on these sites to be generally more reliable.

Libraries

The widespread use of the Internet has led to libraries' Web sites having become more and more powerful and diverse in the functions offered, going beyond searching library indexes, and now providing a range of other services.

Schools

There are many schools of Chinese medicine which teach and conduct research on Chinese medicine, and as a result their Web sites usually offer much information about Chinese medicine. This chapter lists the Web sites of schools of Chinese medicine, both in China and in Western countries.

Journals

This chapter lists journals of Chinese medicine and CAM journals which can found on the Internet, including academic journals and newsletters. Online newsletters usually are free. Journals offer the best source for an understanding of the newest developments and research results.

Databases

Web sites of databases/bibliographies and electronic texts are re-search-oriented tools, and intended for researchers, librarians, and faculties.

History and Philosophy

It is necessary for students of Chinese medicine to study its history. The history of Chinese medicine is like a key to open the door to its treasures. In this chapter, useful and often well-known Web sites are listed that focus on the history of Chinese medicine. This chapter also lists and introduces Chinese medical classics that are available online—with some able to be downloaded at no charge—since learning from the medical classics is the most important way to understanding Chinese medical theories and experiences.

The number of Web sites on Chinese medicine is abundant, but how to use these Web sites effectively and wisely for research and education remains a great challenge in the future.[59]

ASSUMPTIONS

1. This book is for an English-speaking readership but it is un-avoidable that the links to many Web sites will be written in Chinese, and even in Japanese.
2. This book does not discuss online information on hospital, publisher, Tibetan medicine, or Traditional Chinese Veterinary Medicine.
3. This guide is not meant to be an introduction to the Internet itself. The book assumes that the reader has a working knowl-edge of Web browsers, and is able to use search engines and databases.

4. The medical methods and treatments mentioned in this book are not intended to help a reader diagnose, treat, cure, or prevent any disease. If the reader wants to use Chinese medicine in the treatment of any illness, please consult a qualified doctor or professional expert. NCCAM and ChinesemedicineSampler. com[60] have developed a set of questions to help a reader select a reliable practitioner or acupuncturist.

NOTES

1. http://nccam.nih.gov/news/report.pdf.

2. Herring, S.D. (2001). Using the World Wide Web for research: Are faculty satisfied? *The Journal of Academic Librarianship, 27*(3): 213-219.

3. Molassiotis, Alexander et al. (2004). Quality and safety issues of Web-based information about herbal medicines in the treatment of cancer. *Complementary Therapies in Medicine 12*(4): 217–27.

4. Stirling, Dale (2004). Complementary and alternative medicine: A checklist of online resources. *Online Information Review 28*(1): 43-52. Brazin, Lillian (2003). *The Guide to Complementary and Alternative Medicine on the Internet,* Binghamton, NY: The Haworth Press. Rees, Alan (2001). *The Complementary and Alternative Medicine Information Source Book,* Westport: Oryx Press.

5. Fogelman, Betsy (1993). *The Oriental Medicine Resource Guide: An Information Resource Guide,* Santa Fe: In Word Press. Hu, Bin et al. (eds.) (2006). *Zhong yi yao wen xian jian suo* (Chinese medical literature search), Shanghai: Shanghai Science and technology Press. The purpose of this book is to teach students of Chinese medicine how to search medical terms, databases, dictionaries and documents but the book does not focus on online resources and does not provide ample useful Web sites.

6. National Center for Complementary and Alternative Medicine URL: http://nccam.nih.gov/.

7. Philadelphia College of Osteopathic Medicine URL: http://www .pcom.edu/library/Internet_Guides/Complementary_Information_Reso/ Complementary_&_Comp.html.

8. Medical Subject Healings of National Medical Library URL: http:// www.nlm.nih.gov/mesh/.

9. Eisenberg, David et al. (1993); Eisenberg, David et al (1998).

10. The Alternative Medicine Homepage URL: http://www.pitt.edu/ ~cbw/altm.html.

11. *The Oxford Concise Medical Dictionary* (5th ed.) (1998). Oxford: Oxford University Press, pp. 20,142.

12. *The Oxford Concise Medical Dictionary* (6th ed.) (2002). Oxford: Oxford University Press, pp. 22 & 150.

13. Actually, CAM is not always complementary to Western medicine. It may be used independently.

14. Angell, Marcia and Kassirer, Jerome (1998). Alternative medicine: The risks of untested and unregulated remedies. *New England Journal of Medicine 339*(12): 839-841.

15. Wetzel, MS et al. (1998). Courses involving complementary and alternative medicine at US medical schools. *Journal of the American Medical Association, 280:* 784-787. Vickery, Connie E et al. (2006). Complementary and Alternative Medicine Education in Dietetics Programs: Existent but Not Consistent, *Journal of the American Dietetic Association 106*(6): 860-866.

16. Stanford University CAM Program URL: http://camps.stanford .edu/.

17. UBC Medical Library URL: http://toby.library.ubc.ca/subjects/ subjpage1.cfm?id = 234. McMaster University URL: http://hsl.mcmaster .ca/tomflem/altmed.html.

18. Oregon Center for Complementary and Alternative Medicine in Neurological Disorders URL: http://www.ohsu.edu/orccamind/about .shtml. Columbia University, The Richard and Hinda Rosenthal Center for Complementary and Alternative Medicine URL: http://cait.cpmc.columbia .edu:88/dept/rosenthal/About_us.html.

19. What is CAM <http://nccam.nih.gov/health/whatiscam/>.

20. Wikipedia. <en.wikipedia.org/wiki/Chinese_medicine> (Accessed 12 September 2006).

21. Harris, R. (1997). Evaluating Internet Research Sources. <www .virtualsalt.com/evalu8it.htm>. How to Evaluate Medical Information Found on the Internet, <new.cmanet.org/publicdoc.cfm/60/0/GENER/99>. Criteria for Assessing the Quality of Health Information on the Internet-Policy Paper. <hitiweb.mitretek.org/docs/policy.html>. How To Evaluate Health Information on the Internet: Questions and Answers. <www.cancer.gov/ cancertopics/factsheet/Information/internet>. Kovacs, Diane K et al. (2000). *How to Find Medical Information on the Internet: A Print and Online Tutorial for the Healthcare Professional and Consumer,* Berkeley: Library Solutions Press.

22. Lillian Brazin, *Guide to Complementary and Alternative Medicine on the Internet.* Binghamton, NY: The Haworth Press. pp. 6-7.

23. See How to Evaluate Medical Information Found on the Internet. <www.cmanet.org/publicdoc.cfm/60/1/GENER/99>.

24. Sinomedicine is a very strange term, and only used in this book. About introduction to TCM, may also see PC Leung et al. (eds.), *A Comprehensive Guide to Chinese Medicine* (Singapore: World Scientific Co, 2003). Zhang, Yu Huan et al. (1999). *Who Can Ride the Dragon? An Exploration of the Cultural Roots of Traditional Chinese Medicine,* Brookline: Paradigm Publications. Maciocia, Giovanni (2005). *The Foundations of Chinese Medicine: A Comprehensive Text for Acupuncturists and Herbalists,* Edinburgh: Elsevier Churchill Livingstone.

25. Wiseman, Nigel and Feng Ye (1998). *A Practical Dictionary of Chinese Medicine,* Brookline: Paradigm Publication, p. 5.

26. Ibid., p.5.

27. Ibid., p.6.

28. Chu, Joe Hing Kowk. Chinese medical classics. <alternativehealing .org/list_of_Chinese_medical_classics.htm#Ben%20Cao%20Gang%20Mu>.

29. Shuai, Xue Zhong et al (eds) (2006). *Terminology of Traditional Chinese Medicine,* Changsha: Hunan Science & Technology Press, p. 64.

30. Wiseman and Fe, p.106.

31. Yang, Xinrong (ed.) (2003). *Traditional Chinese Medicine: Symptoms, therapy and herbal remedies: A manual from A-Z,* Berlin: Springer, p. 151.

32. Wiseman and Fe, p. 169.

33. Ibid., p. 171.

34. Ibid., p. 204.

35. Shuai, Xue Zhong et al. (eds.), p. 8.

36. Ibid., p. 225.

37. Ibid., p. 226.

38. Ernst, Edzard et al. (eds.) (2006). *The Desktop Guide to Complementary and Alternative Medicine,* Edinburgh: Mosby Elslvier, p. 319.

39. Wikipedia-Huangdi neijing. <en.wikipedia.org/wiki/Huangdi_ Neijing> (accessed at 16 Jan 2007).

40. Wiseman and Fe, p. 389.

41. Zhang, Qiwen et al. (ed.) (2001). *A Practical Chinese-English Dictionary of Traditional Chinese Medicine,* Jinan: Shandong Science and Technology Press, pp. 562-563.

42. Wiseman and Fe, p. 324.

43. Gascoigne, Stephen (1997). *The Chinese way to health: A self-help guide to Traditional Chinese Medicine,* Boston: Tuttle Publishing, p. 48.

44. Wiseman and Fe, p. 402.

45. Zhang, Qiwen et al. (ed.), pp. 562-563.

46. Shuai, Xue Zhong et al. (eds.), p. 61.

47. Wiseman and Fe, pp. 477-478.

48. Fan, Jian Min. *Shang Han Lun and The Golden Chamber.* <www
.pacificcollege.edu/alumni/newsletters/summer2001/shang_hun_lun
.html>.

49. Zhang, Qiwen Zhang et al. (ed.), p. 776.

50. Wiseman and Fe, pp. 313 & 526.

51. Ibid, p. 535.

52. Ernst, Edzard et al. (eds.), p. 352.

53. WHO <www.who.int/medicines/areas/traditional/en/>.

54. Wiseman and Fe, p. 387.

55. Ibid, p. 658.

56. Shuai, Xue Zhong et al. (eds.), p. 1.

57. Wiseman and Fe, p. 49.

58. China Academy of Chinese Medical Sciences (ed.) (1996). *Chinese
traditional medicine and materia medica subject headings,* Beijing: *Zhong
yi gu ji chu ban she.*

59. Recently, the techniques of knowledge management and knowledge
discovery are applied in handling resources of Chinese medicine. Lai,
Iat Long Alex (2005). Knowledge management for Chinese medicines: a
conceptual model, *Information Management & Computer Security 13*(3):
244-255. Feng, Yi et al. (2006). Knowledge discovery in Traditional Chinese Medicine: State of the art and perspectives, *Artificial Intelligence in
Medicine 38*(3): 219-236.

60. ChinesemedicineSampler.com <www.chinesemedicinesampler.com/
chooseintro.html>.

Chapter 1

Portals and General Web Sites

To many Western audiences, acupuncture and Qigong are the symbolic icons of Traditional Chinese Medicine. In fact, beyond these facets of the traditional Chinese medical system are theories and practices that are inseparable from other branches of Chinese culture. Among all branches of cultural learning, religions and philosophy have deeply influenced the development of Chinese medicine. Undoubtedly, knowing more about Chinese history and culture would be advantageous to learning Chinese medicine. In addition, the Romanization of Chinese characters in Mandarin pronunciation, the Pinyin system, should not be neglected by anyone who is interested in any subjects of Chinese culture.

Web sites selected in this chapter provide useful TCM-related information at different levels and for different purposes. There are Web sites that offer useful periodic news, and those that present detailed descriptions of Chinese medical concepts. They are established by government authorities, private institutions, or even individuals. One of the selecting criterion is that these Web sites are informational in specific aspects. Readers should review the Web sites carefully before employing the information.

GENERAL CHINESE CULTURE

Asia Resources on the World Wide Web
http://www.aasianst.org/asiawww.htm
English

> One section in the newsletter lists online resources related to Asian studies. The contents include a valuable list of annotated links.

Asian Studies WWW Monitor
http://coombs.anu.edu.au/asia-www-monitor.html
English

> Established in 1994, the Web site offers abstracts and reviews of updated online resources which are important to research and teaching of Asian Studies. The Web site provides an invaluable service, and it is updated almost daily, with reliable evaluations of each resource's content and research value.

Association for Asian Studies
http://www.aasianst.org/
English

> The association, the most significant society in the field of Asian studies, aims to increase scholars' and interested persons' understanding of East, South, and Southeast Asia, through its journal, newsletter, annual meeting, and numerous seminars. The Web site introduces its structure, annual meetings, published matters, including introductions on and the tables of contents of the *Journal of Asian Studies* and *Education About Asia*.

European Association for Chinese Studies
http://www.soas.ac.uk/eacs/
English

> The association, an important organization in the field of Chinese studies in Europe, aims to promote all scholarly activi-

ties, publishes free online newsletter, and to offer news of conferences, seminars, and scholarship. It also has a database of sinological serials in European libraries. The Web site mainly introduces the European Association for Chinese Studies, its structure, library, and published matters.

International Institute for Asian Studies
http://www.iias.nl/
English

The institute, focusing on human and social sciences, is a postdoctoral research center based in Leiden University, the Netherlands. Its purpose is to promote the interdisciplinary and comparative study of Asia and to encourage international cooperation in the field of Asian studies.

Internet Guide for China Studies
http://sun.sino.uni-heidelberg.de/igcs/
English

This is a carefully selected and annotated resource. The Web site is created and regularly updated by Hanno Lecher, a librarian at the University of Heidelberg. The page makes a very good Internet resources guide.

Pinyin.Info-A Guide to the writing of Mandarin Chinese
**   in Romanization**
http://pinyin.info/index.html
English

This Web site provides a better understanding of the Chinese languages and how Romanization can be used to write Chinese characters. Through providing many readings and publications, Pinyin Info teaches about Romanization of Chinese characters. The site provides sample chapters of selected books about Chinese Romanization and Romanization tool, and it introduces Pinyin rule.

Taoism Information page
http://www.religiousworlds.com/taoism/index.html
English

> The Web site introduces Taoism. Taoist philosophy is closely related to Chinese medicine. A better understanding of Taoist philosophy will make understanding Chinese medical concepts easier. The Web site provides links to pages on acupuncture and martial arts.

TRADITIONAL CHINESE MEDICINE

A-Z of TCM, the Asanté Academy of Chinese medicine
http://www.asante-academy.com/a-z-tcm.htm
English

> The Web site introduces the different elements of Chinese medicine. It is divided into several columns: Ailments and Treatments A to Z examines Western medical conditions from a TCM perspective and gives a brief explanation of how a Traditional Chinese physician would deal with these conditions; Theory and Philosophy A to Z gives brief definitions and explanations of some of the main concepts and terms used in Traditional Chinese Medicine; Medicines A to Z gives an introduction to various herbs and herbal formulae, including their ingredients, functions, and indications; and Foods A to Z gives brief definitions and explanations of everyday foods, and how they can be used to benefit and to maintain health in the theory of Traditional Chinese Medicine.

A Brief Discussion on TCM
http://lulala.ca/tcm/index.html
Chinese (traditional)

> The Web site introduces the origin, development, characteristics, main contents, and modern progress of Traditional Chinese Medicine.

An Expatiation on Traditional Chinese Medicine
http://cmedicine.org/
Chinese (traditional)

> The Web site introduces TCM knowledge, ways of healing and life nourishing, therapeutic diet, medical herbs, and TCM classics. The contents are mainly common knowledge accompanied by interesting stories.

Ancient Way
http://www.ancientway.com/index.html
English

> Although the Web site is constructed for commercial purpose, it has detailed introductions on TCM, acupuncture, massage, and Qigong.

Asia-Pacific TCM Network
http://www.aptcm.com/APTCM/AptcmIndex.html
Chinese (traditional)

> The Web site provides links to Traditional Chinese Medicine online resources according to categories, which includes governmental departments, hospitals and clinics, civil organizations, academic research, herbal production and marketing, education and learning, academic units, journals and magazines, companies, acupuncture and massage, and other alternative therapies. The Web site also collects news regarding the herbal market in China.

Baimu Medicine
http://www.100md.com/index/0L/
Chinese (simplified)

The Web site provides loads of TCM information. The contents of the page includes news, knowledge, books, academic papers, Chinese pharmacology, acupuncture, TCM culture, science research and education, etc. The information is rich, and every column is equipped with many articles related to the topic. Though the information is free, many of the articles can be downloaded and viewed only with a paid registration. The section "Traditional Medicine" is further divided under topics like "basics of Traditional Chinese Medicine," "theory examination," "Traditional Chinese Medicine treatment," "Traditional Chinese Medicine diagnosis," "the integration of Chinese and Western medicine" and introductions on Chinese pharmacology, patented medicine and formulae. Nonetheless, all items are only available to registered users. In terms of the number of topics, the content is rich.

Beijing TCM Education Online
http://210.77.146.154:8080/iTCMedu/bj/index.jsp
Chinese (simplified)

The Web site provides news of Beijing TCM Education. Once registered, visitors can view all TCM educational materials on the Web site. The materials cover a broad range of topics like TCM basic theory, clinical TCM, specialists, and the integration of Chinese and Western medicines. The Web site also covers news and achievement of TCM scientific research in Beijing area, with introductions to TCM hospitals and experts.

Beijing TCM Information Portal
http://www.bjtcm.gov.cn/
Chinese (simplified)

Maintained by the Traditional Chinese Medicine Authority of the city of Beijing, the Web site provides TCM news, policies, and legal documents, scientific research and education in Beijing. It introduces famous physicians in Beijing, governmental units, and services.

Bioon.com
http://www.bioon.com/Article/ShowClass.asp?ClassID = 222
Chinese (simplified) and English

It is indeed a huge medical Web site that has a section on TCM. The contents include TCM basics, practitioners' experience sharing, TCM classics, TCM discussion and thinking, other traditional medicine, formulae, history of Chinese medicine, clinical TCM, TCM news, activities, and pictures. The Web site provides plenty of TCM classics in full text. Some titles can be read only after registration, and others are free of charge. All information and articles provided by the Web site can be read for free. The Web site is also available in English; however, it carries less content than its Chinese counterpart. It has sections "Chinese HerbInfo List," "Organization," "Enterprise," "Market," and "Research."

Calm Spirit Healthcare Online
http://www.calmspirit.com
English

The site has the following sections: "application of Chinese medicinals," "*Tui na* Chinese remedial massage," "*Tui na* general prevention massage," "translations from Chinese Medical texts" and "Qigong." The content is brief.

CAM-Cancer
http://www.cam-cancer.org/
English

Funded under the European Commission 5th Framework Program, the Web site actually is a product of a project titled "Concerted Action for Complementary and Alternative Medicine assessment in the Cancer field." It aims to offer reliable information on complementary and alternative medicines relating to cancer care. The Web site provides studies on acupuncture and cancer.

China Care Net of Traditional Chinese Medicine
http://www.usetm.com/big5/
Chinese (traditional)

The Web site collects TCM news, with its emphasis on disease treatment. Its content covers internal medicine, gynecology, pediatrics, otorhinolaryngology, oncology, clinical research, TCM theory, healthy diet, and herbal medicine. Most reports are short and precise.

China, Chi, and Chicanery: Examining Traditional Chinese
    Medicine and Chi Theory
http://www.csicop.org/si/9509/chi.html#author
English

The page is in fact an essay that was published on *Skeptical Inquirer.* The essay introduces the concept of "middle energizer" in Traditional Chinese Medicine.

China Chief Medical Net: TCM
http://www.shouxi.net/zhongyi/
Chinese (simplified)

This is the TCM section of the Web site "China Chief Medical Net." Its includes herbalist news, a list of forty-eight acupoints attached with illustrations, a detailed description of 116 kinds of herbal medicine, a discussion on sixty-two TCM prescriptions, and an introduction to six famous physicians. Selected contents from the electronic journal published by the Web site can be read online for free.

China TCM Education Online
http://big5.itcmedu.com/
http://gb.itcmedu.com/
http://english.itcmedu.com/
Chinese (traditional and simplified) and English

The establishment of the Web site is mainly for TCM education. The Web site provides information about TCM courses, physician licensing examinations, and related news. The contents include TCM news, TCM school admission news, practitioner laws and morals, TCM education news, and links to TCM online resources.

China TCM Web
http://www.cn939.com/en/index.htm
Chinese (simplified) and English

The Web site offers comprehensive information on Chinese medicine. It contains "Main Page," "DiseaseEncyclopedia," "TCM-News," "AdviceFromDoctor," "DietTherapy," "TCM-Health-Wellness," "SexualHealth," "HealthColumn," "Special-featured therapy," "ChineseHerbs," "TCM-Acupuncture" and "TCM-Tuina."

The pages are very difficult to download. The Chinese version covers more detailed information than the English one.

Chinese Herb Garden
http://healther.stormloader.com/
English

The contents of the Web site is the English version of *Zhong yi de ke xue yuan li* (Scientific Reasons of Chinese Medicine) by

Chen Hua. It has a chapter on Outline of Sinomedicine, which covers the yin-yang theory, the five elements theory, the zangfu theory, the jing luo theory, etiology, the diagnostics, therapeutics of drugs, the drugs and prescriptions; another chapter on the Scientific Principle of Sinomedicine, which explains yin and yang, the five elements and drugs and prescriptions from a scientific perspective; a chapter on Secret Recipes of Sinomedicine, which describes the diseases of digestive system, diseases of urinary system, diseases of circulatory system and blood, diseases of endocrine system, diseases of reproductive system, diseases of skeletal system and muscular system, tumors and cancers, and diseases of skin.

Chinese Herbal Medicine Healthy Information Portal
http://nricm2.nricm.edu.tw/
Chinese (traditional)

This Web site is an information network that lists relevant links according to topics. The topics include: "history of Traditional Chinese Medicine," "Chinese physician's ways of diagnosing," "acupuncture," "healthy diet," "Qigong," "life nourishing," and many others. Also, there is a database on the theories of channels (meridians) and collaterals, one on herbology, and one on formulae. Moreover, it announces news in the field of Traditional Chinese Medicine in Taiwan.

Chinese Medicine and Acupuncture in Canada
http://www.medicinechinese.com/
English

The Web site has a precise introduction on TCM theories and therapies. The section "What is TCM?" introduces the history and basic principles behind TCM, which includes yin-yang theory, the Five Elements theory, vital substances, meridians and channels, zangfu, causes of disharmony, and TCM diagnosis. It also talks about various types of treatment, like acupuncture, herbology, Tui na, Qigong and dietotherapy. The Web site lists

TCM practitioners in Canada, schools and professional associations, government regulations, and suppliers.

Chinese Medical Basics
http://www.theqi.com/cmed/cmed_top.html
Chinese (traditional)

This Web site is an introduction to Traditional Chinese Medicine. It covers basic concepts (including yin-yang theory, five element theory, zangfu theory, jing luo theory, etiologic factors, diagnostic methods, pattern identification, prevention, the five movements and six qi and dietotherapy); a survey on medical herbs (includes herbal medicine, a brief table of Chinese herbs, pattern identification and choice of medicine, verses of formulae, index of formulae and life nourishing Chinese medicine); a summary of every specialty, ancient classics, and terminologies. Overall, the Web site describes Traditional Chinese Medicine in detail. Among all information, the brief table of Chinese herbs, the ancient classics and the terminologies are the most useful references.

Chinese Medicine Sampler
http://www.chinesemedicinesampler.com/
English

The Web site introduces the theory of TCM, diagnosis, herbal medicine, acupuncture, what TCM treats, and provides a pathology guide.

Dave's Psoriasis Information
http://www.psorsite.com/tcm.html
English

The site collected information about Traditional Chinese Medicine treating psoriasis.

EChinaherbs
http://www.echinaherbs.com/2004/index.asp
Chinese (simplified) and English

> The Web site reports TCM news. It introduces TCM life nourishing, dietary, and medical formulae. There is a list of TCM practitioners as well. The English version has different contents, which are categorized into "news," "life," "Chinese medicine therapy," "SARS roundup," "Chinese Medicated Diet," *Huangdi neijing*, "Rehabilitation by Psychotherapy" and "Rehabilitation with Diet."

Famous and Prominent Doctors in Traditional Chinese
   Medicine in China Portal
http://www.famousdoctorstcm.org/default.aspx
Chinese (simplified and traditional) and English

> The Web site is maintained by the World Federation of Chinese Medicine Societies and the Tung Wah Group of Hospitals, Hong Kong. It focuses on introducing famous physicians in Chinese history and of modern times in Mainland China. Visitors can search for physicians in Mainland China by organization, specialty, or regions. The Web site has news, an herbal dictionary, and information about TCM in Hong Kong. The herbal dictionary houses 223 entries with illustrations and a search engine.

The Five Organ Network of Chinese Medicine
http://www.itmonline.org/5organs/5organs.htm
English

> The Web site introduces the five organs: heart, liver, spleen, lung, and kidney, and their functions. Its contents include "Views from the Past" that is some translation of ancient texts, "Properties and Functions," "Pathogenesis," "Basic Guidelines for the Treatment," "Typical Disease Pattern," etc.

Five Element Acupuncture Information Site
www.5element.com.au
English

> Five Element Acupuncture is one form of acupuncture. The Web site introduces Five Element Acupuncture. Its contents include "acupuncture," "five elements," "the twelve meridians," "history of five element," "acupuncture points," and "articles."
>
> If you want to know more about five elements in Chinese culture, please see the URL: http://weber.ucsd.edu/~dkjordan/chin/hbwuushyng.html

Gancao.net
http://gancao.net/
English

> The Web site provides much research on TCM therapy that can be viewed online. "Forum" acts as a platform for practitioners to discuss TCM. "AcuLinks WWW Directory" lists links to TCM-related Web sites for consumers, students, and practitioners. Currently, over 600 unique links, all Web sites with information in depth and of quality, were presented on the list. "Acublog: Western Research, Eastern Medicine" reinterprets biomedical research through a traditional Chinese medical perspective.

Guizhou Modernization of TCM Information Network
http://www.gzyy.org/
Chinese (simplified)

> The Web site reports news about TCM in Guizhou province, especially on the supply of medicinal materials and about the research on TCM modernization. Also, it introduces newly developed medicine.

Guizhou TCM Education Online
http://210.77.146.154:8080/iTCMedu/gzzx/index.jsp
Chinese (simplified)

The Web site provides news about TCM education in Guizhou province. It also covers results and news of TCM research in Guizhou, along with introductions to TCM hospitals and experts, and documents of TCM policy.

Han-Tang TCM Net
http://www.chinesemedicines.net/
Chinese (simplified)

The site provides dictionaries of Chinese medical terms and Chinese medicinal, searched by keyword and strokes of a Chinese character.

Hua Xia Traditional Chinese Medicine
http://www.98800.net/
Chinese (simplified)

The Web site provides abundant articles and the latest information on Traditional Chinese Medicine. The registration is free. Once registered, visitors can download medical classics, e.g., *Wai ke zheng zong* (Orthodox external medicine).

Hulu TCM Professorial Web site
http://www.hulu.com.tw/
Chinese (traditional)

The Web site mainly introduces Chinese medical herbs. It provides TCM articles which cover broad topics including Traditional Chinese Medicine, Chinese pharmacology, therapy, and dietotherapy. The highlight of the Web site is its introduction to over 2,500 kinds of herbal plants, all attached with pictures.

Hunan TCM Online
http://210.77.146.154:8080/iTCMedu/hnzx/index.jsp
Chinese (simplified)

The site mainly provides Chinese medical information of Hunan Province, including hot issues, education, articles, and administration.

Introduction to Glossary of Chinese Medical Terms and
Acupuncture Points
http://www.paradigm-pubs.com/sites/www.paradigm-pubs
.com/files/files/glchme-text.pdf
English

The site is a long article discussing the method and rules for the glossary, which includes Chinese medical terms and names of acupuncture points. A very useful introduction, especially on the English translation of Chinese medical terms.

Jiangsu TCM Information Portal
http://www.jstcm.com/
Chinese (simplified)

The Web site reports news of Traditional Chinese Medicine in Jiangsu province. Its section on "TCM academic" introduces famous physicians in Jiangsu province, TCM documents, a discussion on TCM development and TCM culture. The Web site also makes classics like *Shang han lun, Wen re lun* (On Warm Heat), *Shennong bencao jing* available for downloading, along with free online contents of its journal, *Jiangsu TCM News*. Another section is titled "TCM Exam," which is established for the discussion of Traditional Chinese Medicine and TCM physicians licensing examination.

Medboo TCM and Acupuncture
http://www.ontcm.com/
English

> The information on the Web site is categorized into: "Training
> Program," "Disease Special," "Herbs Garden" that is further
> divided into "Common Herb," "Herb Collection," "Herb Prepa-
> ration" and "Herb Cooking," "Healthy Living" that is further
> divided into "Healthy Foods," "Qigong" and "Taiji," "Acupunc-
> ture" that is further divided into "Basic Theories" and "Clinical
> Reports," "TCM Culture" and "Organizations."

Medical Education Web: TCM Canon
http://www.med66.com/web/zhongyi/
Chinese (simplified)

> TCM Canon is part of the Medical Education Web. It compre-
> hensively introduces TCM knowledge, including basic concepts,
> diagnosis and therapy, health care, cosmetology, jing luo theory,
> biographies of famous physicians, prescriptions, and TCM il-
> lustration.

Michael Tierra's East West Herb Course and Planetary Herbs
    and Formulas
http://www.planetherbs.com/showcase/
English

> The most important part of the site is the section "Articles,"
> which has many TCM-related articles.

Nanyang Zhang Zhongjing TCM Information Portal of China
http://www.zhongjing.net.cn/
Chinese (simplified)

> The Web site is named after Zhang Zhongjing, the author of
> *Shang han lun*. It discusses TCM culture, TCM laws, famous
> physicians, selection of herbs, empirical formulae, and TCM
> classics. It includes the original texts from classics like *Huangdi*

neijing, Nan jing, Shang han lun, Qian jin fang (Prescriptions worth a thousand gold for emergencies, written by Sun Simiao of Tang dynasty). The section "TCM culture" deals with the development and history of Traditional Chinese Medicine, and the section "empirical formulae" introduces prescriptions for common illnesses.

Open Directory Project-Acupuncture and Chinese medicine
http://dmoz.org/Health/Alternative/Acupuncture_and_
  Chinese_Medicine/
English

It provides links to Web sites on "Acupuncture and Chinese medicine," which are divided into "practitioners," "professional organizations," "publications," "schools," "acupuncture," "bodywork," "books," "Chinese herbal medicine," "professional supplies," and "qigong." A brief introduction comes with every link. It links to Web sites in Dutch, French, German, Italian, Japanese, Russian, Swedish, etc.

Orient Medicine
http://www.medizone.com.cn/html/1843.htm
Chinese (simplified)

It links to TCM Web sites with brief descriptions.

Oriental Medicine
http://www.orientalmedicine.com/
English

The Web offers detailed, useful, and updated information on Oriental Medicine, including its philosophies, modalities, strengths, and weaknesses. The contents of the Web site include general information, basic theory, syndromes differentiation, acupuncture, herbal medicine, meditation, and disorders. Each of these sections explains basic theories in detail.

The Pulse of Oriental Medicine
http://www.pulsemed.org/
English

> This is a Web site constructed by Brian B. Carter. It is divided into three sections: "Acupuncture and Oriental Medicine," "Chinese Herbs," and "Diseases and Conditions." In each section, there are news, introductory articles and other information. Visitors can sign up for a free health newsletter, *eZine*.

Reference.com
http://www.reference.com/Dir/Health/Alternative/
  Acupuncture_and_Chinese_Medicine
English

> The site provides links to Chinese medicine and acupuncture with brief description.

References Materials, Paradigm Publications
http://www.paradigm-pubs.com/resources/reference
English

> Paradigm Publications is a press that specializes in publishing books on Chinese medicine. In this Web site, many scholars, including Nigel Wiseman, Eric Brand, Stephen Birch, Robert Felt, Paul U. Unschuld, Marnae Ergil, Z'ev Rosenberg, Yoshio Manaka, Kazuko Itaya, Edward Schafer, Bob Flaws, and Sonya Pritzker, provide their articles. These articles are very useful and practical. For example, Nigel Wiseman offers over ten articles on the discussion of English translation of Chinese medical terms. Paul U. Unschuld offers his New Sources on the History of Chinese Medicine and Chinese Medicine: Nature Versus Chemistry and Technology.

Review of Chinese Medicine
http://japan.ucsd.edu/marta/resources/chinesemed/
  chinesemed.html
English

The page is maintained by Angie Ng. It offers selected links with annotation to Chinese medicine.

Robert Helmer's Web site
http://www.roberthelmer.ca/index.html
English

The page is maintained by Robert Helmer. It features his essays on TCM therapies treating bedwetting, eczema, ear infections, asthma, colic, and on the relationship between TCM and children.

Shandong TCM Information Portal
http://www.sintcm.com.cn/
Chinese (simplified)

The Web site focuses on the information and laws of TCM practices in the Shandong province. The Web site was still under construction when the author browsed it.

Tao of Healing
http://www.geocities.com/HotSprings/2426/
English

The Web site introduces Taoism, Traditional Chinese Medicine and the relationship between the two. The sections of the Web site include "Answers to a Few Basic Questions," "The Nine Taoist Healing Arts," "Chinese Medicine and Breast Cancer," and "Herbal Training Formulas in the Taoist Tradition."

TCM and SARS
http://www.cintcm.com/SARS/index.htm
Chinese (simplified)

The purpose of the Web site is to offer news, reports, and links about the relationship between severe acute respiratory syndrome (SARS) and Chinese medicine, especially on treating SARS with Chinese medicine.

TCM Basic
http://www.tcmbasics.com/
English

Maintained by Wyith Institute of Technology and Tyith Incorporated, the Web site has sections named: "Introduction to TCM," "Basics of TCM," "Classification of Antineoplastic Herbal Medicines," "Zang-fu Theories," "Diagnose," "Prescriptions," "Theories of Channels (Meridians) and Collaterals," "Reference: The Modern View of the Immune System," "Differentiation of Syndromes," "Etiology," and "Materia Medica."

TCM Central
http://www.tcmcentral.com/
English

The Web site deals with acupuncture, auricular acupuncture, herbology, TCM theory, pathologies, nutrition, and bodywork. It also posts news about acupuncture news, which announces acupunctural research achievements in the English world.

TCM English Learning
http://www.itcmedu.com/
Chinese (simplified and traditional), English

The Web site provides information of Traditional Chinese Medicine, which covers important news, research updates, journals, and TCM culture. It has articles and documents regarding Chinese government policy on Traditional Chinese Medicine. The journal links to *Beijing Chinese Physician, Distant Modern TCM Education in China,* and *Hunan TCM Journal.* Therefore, not all articles can be read through the Web site. It has a briefing on the TCM licensing examination with selected articles available online.

TCM Famous Practitioners Web
http://www.zhongyimingjia.com/
Chinese (simplified)

The Web site introduces famous TCM practitioners in Mainland China, their literature, their experiences and learning process. The page is updated daily. Many practitioners in China are online to discuss TCM with visitors.

TCM Guide Informational Network
http://www.tcmguide.com/modules/mylinks/
Chinese (traditional)

The Web site is a guiding network that links to other Web sites that deal with TCM education, health care, medical care centers, pharmacies and pharmaceutical companies, universities, document search, commercial services, print and media, and governmental departments.

TCM Online (China TCM Information Network)
http://www.cintcm.com/
http://www.cintcm.ac.cn
Chinese (simplified and traditional), English

The Web site is established by Zhongyanxin Chinese Medicine and Pharmacology Information Network Company in Beijing. It broadcasts news of Traditional Chinese Medicine in Mainland China. The content of the Web site includes, "Databases," "TCM Professional," "Club TCM Forum," "Research," "Online Education," "Directory," "TCM Legislation," "Commerce Information," "BBS," and "Organization." The Web site aims to expand the TCM database. Currently, ten databases are built. These are useful tools for studying Traditional Chinese Medicine. The "Cyclopaedia" gives a comprehensive introduction to TCM, whereas the "Q and A" section shares Chinese physicians' experiences in treating illness. Also, there are indexes of twenty titles of TCM journals on the page. The English version of the Web site is currently under construction, and its content is not as rich as its Chinese counterpart.

TCM Student: The world of Acupuncture and Oriental Medicine
http://www.tcmstudent.com/
English

The Web site archives online articles and news about TCM and acupuncture. Visitors can read the collection through links provided on the Web site. The Web site has entries like "school of TCM," "state of laws," "study tool," "books on TCM," "TCM supplies," "TCM software," "national associations," "Web journal," and "acupuncture theory."

Terms Translation for Chinese Medicine
http://www.paradigm-pubs.com/resources/Translation
English

The Web site posts the essay *Considerations for the Translation of Traditional Chinese Medicine Into English,* which explains what merits notice in translating Chinese medical terms into English.

The Shang han Web
http://www.shanghan.com/
Chinese (simplified)

The Web site specializes on *Shang han* (cold damage). It carries articles on the Internet with a "download center" and an "illustration center." Visitors can download the electronic *Zhongjing Academic Journal* published in the "download center."

The Study and the Traces of Thoughts in the Modernization of the Four Examinations in Traditional Chinese Medicine
http://www.cmu.edu.tw/new/cmic/ccmp/
Chinese (traditional)

This Web site is maintained by Professor Chang Yung-hsien of China Medical University and the Committee on Chinese Medicine and Pharmacy, Department of Health, Executive Yuan of Taiwan. It introduces the Four Examinations (Four Diagnoses): inspection, listening and smelling, inquiry, and palpation, their methods and theories. Studying the four examinations through modern scientific methods provides an objective standard of diagnosis in Chinese medicine. Moreover, not only does the Web site convey its information through words, it also expresses itself through pictures and sound, both exclusive Web features.

Traditional Chinese Medicine
http://www.healthy.net/clinic/therapy/Chinmed/index.asp
English

The contents includes "Understanding Chinese Medicine," "History of Acupuncture and Chinese Medicine," "Diagnosis in Chinese Medicine," "Therapeutic Modalities in Acupuncture and Chinese Medicine," "Therapeutic Programs for Specific Conditions," "Traditional Chinese Medicine Information Center," "Traditional Chinese Medicine Resource Center," "National Institutes of Health Consensus Development Statement," "Traditional Chinese Medicine Schools." The section on TCM knowledge is clearly written, which makes it a very good introduction to TCM. Also, its list of TCM school hyperlinks is very complete.

Traditional Chinese Medicine
http://www.umm.edu/altmed/ConsModalities/
  TraditionalChineseMedicinecm.html
English

> This Web site is maintained by the Medical Center of the University of Maryland. Other than introducing the basic concepts of Traditional Chinese Medicine, it has information like "What should I expect on my first visit?" "What is TCM good for?" "Is there anything I should watch out for?" "How can I find a qualified TCM practitioner?" "supporting research," which are all precisely written and worth attention.

Traditional Chinese Medicine and Acupuncture Health
  Information Organization
http://tcm.health-info.org/
English

> The Web site provides rich information on Traditional Chinese Medicine, including acupuncture, Chinese herbal medicine, herbal formulas, foundation and diagnosis, internal medicine, gynecology, *Tui na* massage, pediatrics, health and seasons, dermatology, gerontology, food cure, special senses, common diseases, Qigong and Taiji, prevention, practitioner search, tests for students, related sites and links. Each mentioned section is further divided into smaller divisions that have detailed explanation attached with illustrations.

Traditional Chinese Medicine and Keeping Health
http://www.tcmhk.com/
Chinese (traditional)

> The Web site focuses on TCM and health. It introduces TCM theories like the Eight Principles and the Four Diagnoses, herbology, acupuncture, and TCM classics. The page is established by Hong Kong TCM practitioners, and is attached with a "List

of Famous Physicians" and "Multi-functional Physician Search Engine."

Traditional Chinese Medicine, Department of Human Service, State Government Department, Victoria, Australia
http://www.health.vic.gov.au/archive/archive2006/chinese/
English

The Web site is an evaluation report on TCM practices in the Victoria region, done by experts hired by Department of Human Service of the Victorian State Government Department of Australia from 1996 to 2001. This report provides information on the TCM workforce in Australia, patient usages of TCM, educational institutions providing training, the risks and benefits of TCM, and the need for regulatory controls over its practice. A complete report can be downloaded for free.

Traditional Chinese Medicine in China
http://www.tcm.cn/
Chinese (simplified)

The is indeed the Web site of China TCM Technology Development and Exchange Center, which is under the State Administration of Traditional Chinese Medicine of the People's Republic of China. The Web site focuses on publishing news about TCM in China, and it introduces highlighted projects of the State TCM Department, newly developed medicine, and research projects under state administration. Other sections of the page are still under construction.

Traditional Chinese Medicine Information Page
http://www.tcmpage.com/
Chinese (traditional) and English

The Web site introduces the history, basic concepts, and essentials of Chinese medicine.

Traditional Chinese Medicine Information Portals
http://www.ccmp.gov.tw/
Chinese (traditional) and English

This is the Web site of the Committee on Chinese Medicine and Pharmacy, Department of Health, Executive Yuan, Taiwan. The contents of the Web site are titled "major events," "Chinese medical association," "GMP pharmaceutical company," "traditional pharmaceutical company," "pharmaceutical," "abstracts," "unified formulas," and "laws and regulations."

Traditional Chinese Medicine—Wikipedia, the free
  encyclopedia
http://en.wikipedia.org/wiki/Traditional_Chinese_medicine
English

Wikipedia is one of the most popular free encyclopedias online. In its entry for "Traditional Chinese Medicine," it includes uses of TCM, TCM theory, TCM diagnostics, TCM treatment techniques, TCM and science, the relationship between TCM and Western medicine, and TCM and animals. Wikipedia has been quoted widely by other Web sites, and its influence should not be underestimated. Many Web sites on Traditional Chinese Medicine are directly linked from this page.

Traditional Chinese Medicine ZJ
http://www.zjtcm.gov.cn/
Chinese (simplified)

The Web site aims to report news on Traditional Chinese Medicine in Zhejiang province. Its contents include "medical organization," "news and announcements," "messages from famous physicians," "subjects and specialties," "TCM culture," "TCM corporate," "external exchange," "law and policy," "educational work" and "scientific research." Overall, it has a well-rounded introduction on Traditional Chinese Medicine.

Traditional Medicine: Definitions WHO
http://www.who.int/medicines/areas/traditional/en/
English (Arabic, simplified Chinese, French, Russian, Spanish
versions are currently unavailable)

The World Health Organization publishes its definitions of traditional medicine terms on this page. It precisely defines terms like "traditional medicine," "alternative and complementary medicine" and "herbal medicine." WHO also posts the articles, "General Guidelines for Methodologies on Research" and "Evaluation of Traditional Medicine," on the page for free public download.

What is Chinese Medicine?
http://chinese-school.netfirms.com/Chinese-medicine.html
English

This Web site is an elementary introduction to Traditional Chinese Medicine. It has sections like "Articles about Chinese medicine," "Diabetes and Chinese Medicine," and "Articles about Alternative medicine."

Nigel A.R. Wiseman
http://memo.cgu.edu.tw/wiseman/
English

Nigel Wiseman is a renowned scholar who published and edited many books about Chinese medicine. He is an expert on the English translation of Chinese medicine. The Web site offers two very useful PDF files entitled *Learner's Character dictionary of Chinese Medicine* and *Introduction to Chinese Medicine,* which can be downloaded for free. The latter one is very precise and is suitable for a beginner. His Web publications, such as *Rationale for the Terminology of Fundamentals of Chinese Medicine: The Case for Literal Translation,* can also be found on the Web site.

Note: More of Nigel Wiseman's publications are also available online. Readers may visit the URL: http://www.paradigm-pubs.com/WisemanWork.

Yin and Yang in Medical Theory
http://academic.brooklyn.cuny.edu/core9/phalsall/texts/
  yinyang.html
English

> The Web site is established to introduce Chinese culture. This chapter is about yin-yang and five elements theories in Traditional Chinese Medicine, which is a translation of *Huangdi neijing,* from a book by Patricia Ebrey.

ACUPUNCTURE

Acumedico
http://www.acumedico.com/
English

> Shmuel Halevi posts his essays on this Web site (most of the articles were initially published in *Journal of Chinese Medicine*). He also provides a free Web-based acupoints database and illustrations of channels and meridians.

Acupoint Codes, Names, Translations and Locations
http://homepage.eircom.net/~progers/pt.htm
English

> The Web site provides details of codes for meridians and acupoints. The sections of "Acupoint details and locations," "Get acupoint Pinyin name for a selected point code," "Get acupoint code for a selected Pinyin name," and "Acupoint formulas," "Lookup codes for channels, vessels and nonchannel points," "Codes for the twelve main Jing-channels," and "Codes for midline vessels (Dumai, Renmai) and other points" are included.

Acupuncture
http://bmj.bmjjournals.com/cgi/content/full/319/7215/973
English

> This is an article published on *British Medical Journal,* by Andrew Vickers and Catherine Zollman. The content is divided into "background," "how does acupuncture work?" "what happens during a treatment?," "therapeutic scope," "safety of acupuncture" and "practitioners."

Acupuncture
http://www.healthy.net/scr/Author.asp?PeoId = 618
English

> The Web site lists forty-two essays on TCM and acupuncture written by George T. Lewith, which discusses acupunctural theories and evaluates the efficacy of acupuncture.

Acupuncture and TCM Links of Vilberto's Home Page
http://acupuncture.8k.com/acupvil.htm
English

> The Web site provides links according to the following categories: "Personal Pages," "Acupuncture Resources Megasites," "Bookstores," "Library," "Scientific Journals," "Softwares," "CD-roms and Videos for TCM," "Institutions and Associations," "Schools and Education," "Herbology," "Hand Acupuncture/Koryo Acupuncture," "Acupressure/Tuina/Massage," "Veterinary Acupuncture," "Miscellany," "Graphics of Acupoints Online," "Qigong," "Wushu," "Taiji," "Pakua," "Hsing-Yi," "Newsgroups and Mailing Lists," "Alternative Medicine in General," "Western Health Science Sites" and "Chinese Culture."

Acupuncture Guide.Com
http://www.acuxo.com/index.asp
English

Acuxo.com collects acupuncture resources on the Internet. Its contents include "Points," with access to images point locations along with their associated meridians; "Abstracts" permits access to hundreds of National Institutes of Health research documents in an easy- to-use search format; each window provides an abstract, author, date, Web address, publications, and much more. All abstracts are from a variety of subject matter in a broad range of acupuncture, done by top researchers from around the world. The site also has "Meridians," which are "arranged to facilitate quick and convenient data regarding all acupuncture points with images"; "Selections" includes information on point combinations. Acuxo has developed an acupuncture database and pictures, specially designed for Palm and Palmpilot.

Acupuncture NHI Consensus Statement
http://www.healthy.net/LIBRARY/Articles/NIH/Report.htm
English

The Web site posts a report on the method and principles of acupuncture by the National Institutes of Health's report on the several topics: "What is the efficacy of acupuncture, compared with placebo or sham acupuncture, in the conditions for which sufficient data are available to evaluate?" "What is the place of acupuncture in the treatment of various conditions for which sufficient data are available, in comparison with or in combination with other interventions (including no intervention)?" "What is known about the biological effects of acupuncture that helps us understand how it works?" "What issues need to be addressed so that acupuncture may be appropriately incorporated into today's health care system?" and "What are the directions for future research?"

Acupuncture Theory—Traditional Chinese Medicine
http://www.yinyanghouse.com/chinesetheory.html
English

The Web site introduces acupunctural theory and therapy comprehensively. The content includes: "Acupuncture Points," which discusses their locations, functions, and categories; "Acupuncture Theory," its foundations and diagnoses; "Acupuncture Treatments," which compares Western and TCM disorders, "Adjunctive Therapies," "Contributed Articles," "Additional Acupuncture Theory Resources," and "Discuss Acupuncture Theory." There is also an introduction to TCM resources: "Find a Practitioner," "Acupuncture Research," "Discussion Forum," "Latest News," and "Health Information."

Acupuncture / Acupressure Internet Resources
http://www.holisticmed.com/www/acupuncture.html
English

Established by the Holistic Medicine Resource Center, the Web site lists Acupuncture/Acupressure-related Internet resources. However, as the author observed, the latest update was on November 17, 2001.

Acupuncture.Com: Gateway to Chinese Medicine, Health and Wellness
http://www.acupuncture.com/
English

The Web site discusses TCM and acupuncture theory and basics in three sections: for patients, for practitioners, and for students, respectively. The content includes: "Chinese Medicine Basics," "Conditions A-Z," "Herbal Remedies," "Self-Healing Qigong/Tuina," "Diet and Nutrition," "Find an Acupuncturist," "Patient Testimonials," "Animal Acupuncture," "Syndromes A-Z," "Herbology," "Education," "Events," "Resources and Supplies," "Research," "Acupuncture Schools," "Book and Product

Reviews," "Reference Library" and "State Laws." The organization also publishes *Points Newsletter.*

AcuTimes
http://www.acutimes.com/
Chinese (simplified)

The Web site collects acupuncture-related research and news. It has rich contents, including news, academic exchange, theory exploration, clinical studies, education, an electronic journal, achievement news, famous acupuncturists, books on acupuncture, acupunctural cases, acupunctural culture, software, special acupuncture and therapy. Any research or news regarding acupuncture can be found on this Web site. Also, it provides articles on acupuncture, which can be read online for free. Another acupuncture database is currently under construction.

American Acupuncture
http://www.americanacupuncture.com/
English

The Web site covers history, information, and resources of acupuncture.

Chinese Acupuncture
http://www.cmu.edu.tw/new/cmic/acu/index.htm
Chinese (traditional)

There are four sections on the Web site: "Channels and meridians theory and acupoints," "Acupunctural methods," "Acupunctural healing" and "Common acupunctural therapy." Each section is attached with illustrations.

Chinese Acupuncture Net
http://www.zhenjiucn.com/
Chinese (simplified)

The Web site introduces basic theories of channels and meridians, acupoints, acupuncture, *tui na,* treatment, herbal medicine, formulae, etc. During the author's visit, only chapters of channels and meridians, acupoints and acupuncture were loaded with information. Other chapters were incomplete. The contents were still under construction.

Circadian Acupuncture
http://www.acupuncture-acupressure-points.com/
English

The Web site is an introduction to acupuncture and circadian acupuncture. The latter, is also called method of *Zi* (midnight) and *Wu* (midday) Irrigation of the Meridians, recorded in ancient acupuncture canons. It also offers introduction on acupuncture theory and basic theory of Chinese medicine.

Denny Wong Acupuncture Clinic
http://dennywong.net/organizations.htm
English

The Web site collects acupuncture-related links, which includes Web sites of journals, schools, online libraries, discussion groups and resources, miscellaneous, international organizations of acupuncture doctors and physicians. One of the sections on the page, "International Acupuncture Professional Titles," lists and defines titles held by acupuncturists, which would help lay people understand their specialties and qualifications. Moreover, this Web site (http://www.acupuncturetoday.com/abc/titlesandabbreviations.php) lists international acupuncture titles and abbreviations. Another Web site (http://www.arthritis.org/conditions/alttherapies/glossary.asp) lists glossaries of health professional titles, which helps those who want to find out the meanings of the titles.

Medical Acupuncture Web Page
http://users.med.auth.gr/~karanik/english/main.htm
English

The Web site is maintained by the Medical School at Aristotle University of Thessaloniki, Greece. It provides links to other Web sites regarding acupuncture, its basic theory, and usage explanation. There is a section on the Web site on the practice of acupuncture in animals, "The Veterinary Acupuncture Page," which aims to provide educational material on acupuncture to veterinarians. The Web site publishes *Web-journal of Acupuncture.*

Super Acupuncture Guide
http://www.superacupunctureguide.com/index.html
English

The Web site sorts links to online acupuncture information into over 200 categories and provides each category with latest news and recommended Web sites. The Web site also offers news and articles.

TCM Acupuncture Information Center
http://www.cmu.edu.tw/new/cmic/www/index.html
Chinese (traditional)

The Web site is set up by China Medical University Hospital of Taiwan. While the author was browsing it, there was only limited information in the sections, "TCM information" and "Chinese herbology." The Web site is still under construction.

The Voices of Acupuncture
http://www.hnzjzs.com/index.asp
Chinese (simplified)

The Web site is established by the Public Acupuncture Laboratory of Hunan TCM College to provide resources for acupunctural education. Its contents are designed for those who aim to learn acupuncture. It introduces acupunctural specialists and acupunctural research news. Most important, it provides a complete acupuncture education program, whose courses include channels and meridians, acupoints, moxibustion, treatment, research progress, exercises, and questions on acupuncture.

HERBAL

Asia-Pacific Chinese Herb Information
http://istcm.aptcm.com/istcmdb/home.nsf
Chinese (simplified)

The Web site provides news of the herbal market in regard to supply and demand. The Web site also introduces the medicinal market in other countries, TCM basic knowledge and ingredients, the indications, and the growing of 500 kinds of Chinese herbs.

China Golden Medicine
http://www.gm.net.cn/gmweb/default.aspx
Chinese (simplified)

The Web site provides news and information regarding medicine and the demand and supply situation in the herbal market.

Chinese Herbal Formula
http://www.emedicinal.com/herbal-forumulas/chinese.php
English

This page is a section of eMedicinal, which discusses Chinese herbal formulae and diseases they treat.

Chinese Herbs Sources Net
http://www.spec-g.com.tw/newherb/
Chinese (traditional)

The Web site is about sources of TCM. Its section, "Places of Origins," lists the production of medicinal materials by province; "Chinese Herbology" lists 671 kinds of Chinese herbs with illustrations and names in Chinese and English, and it also mentions those that are poisonous; "Selections of Compound Prescription" introduces formulae according to their medical uses, with their names in Chinese, English, and Latin, indications, and ingredients; and "Herbology Classics" lists classical texts by dynasties. All 671 kinds of Chinese herbs listed on this Web site are tested for Certificate of Analysis by the Scientific Pharmaceutical Elite Company. Information regarding the tests can be found on the company's URL: http://www.spec-g.com. tw/herbexam/.

Chinese Medicinal GAP Net
http://www.tcmgap.com/
Chinese (simplified)

In 2002, the State (China's government, PRC) Food and Drug Administration announced "Good Agricultural Practice (GAP) for Chinese Crude Drugs (Interim)" (http://www.sfda.gov.cn/ eng). The Web site offers information on GAP for Chinese Medicinal, created by the GAP Association for Chinese Medicinal Materials. It contains "Main News," "Policy Statute," "GAP Research," "GAP Item Application," "Information on Natural

Medicinal worldwide," "Information on Drug market," "Member" and "GAP Discussion Forum."

Chinese Medicinal Herbs
http://www.zyw168.com/
Chinese (simplified)

The Web site provides analyses of medicinal herbs, patent medicines and the medicine market, along with the production and sales profiles of medicinal technology and medicine in Mainland China.

Chinese Medicine Capital Information Portal
http://www.yaoducn.com/
Chinese (simplified)

The Web site is maintained by the Department of Pharmacy of Zhangshu City in Jiangxi province. Not only does it provide information about the herb production industry in Zhangshu city, it also presents news from across the nation, along with analysis of the industry.

Chinese Natural Medicine Information Net
http://www.yczx.gov.cn/
Chinese (simplified)

Maintained by Yangma Town Government of Jiangsu Province, the Web site gives information regarding production and sales of medicinal herbs in town and other news from market.

Chinese Southern Medicinal Herb Information Net
http://sctcm.com/
Chinese (simplified)

The Web site provides news from the medicinal herb industry. It introduces herb production, resource allocation, species and growing, examination, and the demand and supply situation.

Clinical Chinese Medicine
http://aeam.umin.ac.jp/siryouko/
Japanese

The Web site is established by the East Asian Medical Association. It introduces the history of Chinese medicine and its development in Japan. The Web site posts the original texts of *Su wen, Ling shu, Nan jing, Shang han lun, Jin kui yao lue, Shennong bencao jing,* and *Bian Que Cang Gong Zhuan* (Biography of Bianque) online.

Correct and Incorrect Ways of Choosing Herbs
http://www.rmhiherbal.org/a/e.chooshrbs.html
English

The Web site aims to explore how traditional Chinese herbalists chose herbs and create herbal formulas with clinical effectiveness. The Web site discusses how to choose medicinal herbs correctly and what to notice when choosing.

Global Information Hub on Integrated Medicine
http://www.globinmed.com/IMRContent/default.aspx
English

The Web site, created by the Institute for Medical Research Ministry of Health Malaysia, offers Traditional Chinese Medicine Herbs-professional Data (over 129 TCM herbs) and Traditional Chinese Medicine formulae-professional Data (over fifty-two TCM formulae) in alphabetical order.

Herb No1.com
http://www.herbno1.com/html/herb-index.html
Chinese (traditional)

The Web site introduces medicinal herbs in daily uses. Its contents include "Physicians' Discussion on Medicine," "TCM Database" which houses latest news in TCM research, "Medicine and Beauty," "Medicinal Herbs Illustrations," "Treatments for

Common Diseases" and "Therapies." "Medicinal Herbs Illustrations" lists 200 species of medicinal herbs, sorted by medical uses, with their places of origins, uses, indications and how to avoid frauds.

Hong Kong Chinese Materia Medica Standards
http://www.dh.gov.hk/english/main/main_cm/files/vol1/main
  .html
Chinese (traditional) and English

Conducted by the Department of Health, Hong Kong Special Administrative Region, the purpose of Hong Kong Chinese *Materia Medica* Standards is to provide recommendations and references regarding the safety and quality standards for some Chinese herbal medicines commonly used in Hong Kong. The monograph for each Chinese *Materia Medica* is arranged in the following order: names, source, description, identification, tests, extractives, and assay. Hong Kong Chinese *Materia Medica* Standards has completed the first monograph which includes nine Chinese *Materia Medica* in Hong Kong. The contents can be downloaded from the Web site for free. Interested readers may also refer to a review article which is available at URL: http://www.annals.edu.sg/PDF/35VolNo11Nov2006/V35N11 p764.pdf.

Information of Chinese Medicinal Materials
http://www.herbstimes.com/
Chinese (simplified)

Maintained by the Chinese Medicinal Herbs Research Institute of Nanjing Agriculture University, the Web site provides news about medicinal herbs, introduces latest herb growing technology, reports the condition in the market, and discusses the quality examination of herbs.

Information Net for Adverse Drug Reaction (ARD) of Using Chinese Medicinal
http://www.adr.com.cn/default.asp
Chinese (simplified)

The National Center for ADR Monitoring (http://www.cdr.gov. cn/index.jsp) of the (PRC) State Food and Drug Administration is responsible for drug/medical device adverse reaction (adverse event) monitoring. Some provinces (such as Guangzhou, Hunan, Zhejiang, etc.) also established similar centers. Supported by Guangzhou University of Chinese Medicine, the site focuses on reporting adverse drug reaction when using Chinese medicinals. The Web site offers much information on ADR research, news, case studies, and 100 questions of ADR knowledge. Users can use search engine after registration.

Jeremy Ross: Combining Western Herbs and Chinese Medicine
http://www.jeremyross.com/
English

The page owner is the author of *Combining Western Herbs and Chinese Medicine.* The aim of the page is to keep practitioners up to date with information. The resource section contains free downloads such as interviews, research updates, case histories, and herb lists.

Materia Medica—Chinese Herbal Medicine
http://www.cathedralroadclinic.co.uk/herbal.htm
English

The Web site introduces *Materia Medica* and tonic herbs. Its contents include *Materia Medica,* tonic herbs, traditional tonic herbs, tonic herb formulas, treating side effects, formulas for chemotherapy side effects, radiation therapy side effects, and chronic ulcers.

Meili Chinese Pharmacy
http://home.njenet.net.cn/njsf/mei.htm
Chinese (simplified)

The Web site is divided into three sections: Chinese pharmacy can be used to search for more than 400 kinds of Chinese medicinal materials with illustrations according to their medical functions. Second, the formulae directory can be used to search for related formulae by entering the keywords. Third, Chinese medical classics offers free downloadable *Huangdi neijing, Shennong bencao jing, Nan jing, Shang han lun,* and *Jin gui yao lue* in full text. Users can also download the Directory for Formulae for Internal Medicine for free. The directory has included more than 900 formulae and their ingredients.

Pharmnet
http://www.pharmnet.com.cn/tcm/
Chinese (simplified)

The Web site offers the latest information on medicine, such as new drugs, laws and regulations, productions, and FDA news. It has established two databases, one is for searching pharmaceutical products and the other is for pharmaceutical corporations.

PharmTao
http://www.pharmtao.com/Herb/index.htm
Chinese (simplified) and English

The Web site is available in Chinese and English versions. Other than herbal medicine news, the English version provides an introduction to herbs, medicinal herbs–general, preparation of herbs, forms of using herbs, scientific research of herbs, herb-drug interactions, herbal diet, herbs and beauty, literature on herbs (journals on herbal medicine), and integrative medicine. The Chinese version provides the original texts of Chinese herbal medicine classics, for example, *Shennong bencao jing* and *Tang tou ge jue* (Formula in rhyme).

Qualiherb
http://www.herb.com.tw/
Chinese (traditional) and English

The site is divided into the following categories: most news, Chinese herbalism history and introduction, Chinese herbs/ living photos, Chinese herb for osteoporosis, Chinese patent formulas, and Chinese herb and art on the Silk Road.

Resources of Chinese Medicinal
http://www.tcm-resources.org.cn/
Chinese (simplified)

Maintained by the Institute of Medicinal Plant Development of Chinese Academy of Medical Sciences and Peking Union Medical Colleges, the Web site contains "Survey on Resources of Chinese Medicinal," "Medicinal Plant and Animal Cultivation Centers," "Organizations for Protection," "Law and Standard," "Document Center," "Database Center" and "Introduction to the Institute." The site provides very rich information and resources on medicinal plants of TCM, and also introduces its publications on Chinese medicinals.

The English version is under construction.

South West School of Botanical Medicine
http://www.swsbm.com/HOMEPAGE/HomePage.html
English

The Web site provides source books and manuals about medicinal plants, *Materia Medica* and pharmacy. Some contents relevant to Chinese medicine can be read online for free.

State Board of Protection and Evaluation of Medicinal Herb Species
http://www1.zybh.gov.cn/
Chinese (simplified)

The State Board of Protection and Evaluation of Medicinal Herbs Species is an organization set up by the Chinese government for the protection of herbal species. This is the official Web site of the Board and where it posts laws and policies, publishes documents, evaluates the protection, and other relevant information on the protection of herbal species. The Web site provides "Herbal Species Protection Search" and a "Web site Information Search."

The Chinese Herb Academy
http://www.chineseherbacademy.org/
English

The Web site is hosted by the Chinese Herb Academy. It offers TCM-related links and articles, including *Online Herb Study Guide* by Bob Damone and Todd Luger, *Chinese Medical Terms in Chinese, Pinyin and Wiseman (Herbs, Formulas, Patterns), Thinking Critically about Diet* by Paul Bergner and Todd Luger, *Instructional Design and Technology in TCM* by Todd Luger, and *Information on Acupuncture for Patients* also by Luger.

Traditional Chinese and Western Herbal Medicine in Humans and Animals
http://homepage.eircom.net/~progers/herblink.htm
English

The Web site provides links according to the following categories: "Herbal Medicine Databases: Single Herbs, Herbal Medicine Databases: Formulas," "Drug-Drug and Drug-Herb Interactions," "Herbal Medicine Associations," "Groups,"

"Schools," "Societies," "Herbal Medicine E-mail Discussion Lists," "Online Herbal Study Material," "Journal and Distance Learning," "Herbal Supply Companies (Commercial)." The last update was in 2002, and many of the links are lost.

Traditional Chinese Herbal Medicine
http://healthlibrary.epnet.com/GetContent.aspx?token =
    e0498803-7f62-4563-8d47-5fe33da65dd4andchunkiid = 37410
English

The Web site discusses TCM theories and usages. Its contents include: "Overview," "History of Chinese Herbal Medicine," "Principles of Traditional Chinese Herbal Medicine," "Types of Chinese Herbal Remedies," "What Is Chinese Herbal Medicine Used for Today?," "What Is the Scientific Evidence for Traditional Chinese Herbal Medicine?," "Other Uses for Traditional Chinese Herbal Medicine," "How to Choose a Practitioner of Traditional Chinese Herbal Medicine," "Safety Issues" and "References."

Zhonghua bencao quan shu
http://www.zhongyanhui.com
Chinese (simplified)

Part of the Web site is an introduction the series, *Zhonghua bencao quan shu* (*The complete book of Chinese Materia Medica*). The rest of the contents introduces Chinese *Materia Medica,* including documents (with history of *Materia Medica,* hundreds of abstracts, methods for studying these documents, and an introduction on Chinese medicine), illustrations (includes twenty-seven pictures from the *Materia Medica* classics), database (under construction), and an introduction on dietotherapy.

TAIJI AND CHINESE MASSAGE

Aromatherapy, Massage and Chinese Medicine
http://www.positivehealth.com/permit/Articles/Aromatherapy/
  jobaker.htm
English

It briefly introduces aromatherapy, massage, and Chinese medicine.

Chinese Massage
http://www.experiencefestival.com/chinese_massage
English

The Web site offers some articles on Chinese massage.

Chinese Massage Therapy
http://www.planetherbs.com/articles/tuina.html
English

The Web site introduces Chinese massage therapy, its terms, its jing luo theory, which is the basis of Chinese massage, its techniques, and its treatment in practice.

Electronic Resources on Tai Chi
http://www.chebucto.ns.ca/Philosophy/Taichi/other.html
English

The Web site offers links to other pages regarding Taiji.

Tai Chi
http://www.umm.edu/altmed/articles/tai-chi-000361.htm
English

The Web site is established by the Medical Center of the University of Maryland. It explains the basic Taiji principles.

Tai Chi
http://www.tai-chi.com/
English

In the section "Tai Chi Information," the page introduces Taiji, Qigong and Chinese Internal Martial Art. Its contents include "Using Tai Chi Chuan for Meditation," "What is Jin?" "How Can I Find a Good Teacher?" "What Are the Tai Chi Classics?" "What is Qi?" "What is the proper way to breathe while practicing Tai Chi Chuan?" "What is the Dantian?" "What Does The Term 'Relax' Mean in Tai Chi Chuan?" and "How Do I Do It?"

Tai Chi and Qigong
http://www.harthosp.org/IntMed/taichi.htm
English

It briefly introduces Taiji and Qigong.

Tuina (Traditional Chinese Massage)
http://www.chisuk.org.uk/bodymind/whatis/tuina.php
English

The site briefly introduces Tuina and its history.

DIGITAL MUSEUMS

Beijing TCM Online Museum
http://www.tcm-china.info/
Chinese (Simplified)

The museum Web site is divided into "Main Hall," "Medicinal Herbs Hall," "Famous Physicians Hall," "Palace Medical Hall," "Healing Hall," "Education Hall," "Technology Hall," "Life Nourishing Hall," "Shennong Hundred Herbs Hall," and "Digital Collection." Every Hall houses rich content along with animation.

Guangxi TCM University Medicinal Herb Specimen Hall
http://www.gxtcmu.edu.cn/hzzx/zhongyao.htm
Chinese (Simplified)

The Web site introduces the Specimen Hall.

Hong Kong Museum of Medical Sciences
http://www.hkmms.org.hk/
Chinese (Traditional) and English

The Web site introduces Chinese medicinal herbs housed in the museum's herbal garden.

Museum of Acupuncture
http://iam.acutimes.com/museum_build.asp?class =
109&liststate = 0&ID = 1176
Chinese (Simplified)

It is the Web site of a museum that collects "The bronze human model for acupuncture," "Classics on the bronze human model for acupuncture" and "Chart for acupuncture."

Museum of Materia Medica, University of Toyama
http://www.inm.u-toyama.ac.jp/mmmw/index.html
English and Japanese

The Web site introduces the Museum Materia Medica in the Institute of Natural Medicine, University of Toyama. It is actually an ethnomedicine database that includes both general and scientific information of the samples of *Materia Medica,* stored in the Museum.

TCM Digital Museum
http://bwg.bjucmp.edu.cn/
Chinese (Simplified)

Set up by Beijing TCM University, the Web site is divided into "Introduction to the Museum," "History of Chinese Medicine," and "History of Chinese Pharmacology." The contents are rich and comprehensive. The Web site covers medical appliances, famous physicians in history, ancient medical classics, history of the development of specialties and the history of East-West medicine exchange.

Chapter 2

Organizations

The Web sites in this chapter mainly introduce their respective organizations and publish news relevant to their specific fields. Some of them provide a newsletter, journals, or news. The following are mainly written according to the self-descriptions offered by the organizations online. Any additional information to be noticed will be noted. In the United States, every state has its association or committee for Oriental medicine or acupuncture.

CHINESE MEDICINE, TRADITIONAL MEDICINE, AND ORIENTAL MEDICINE

American Association of Acupuncture and Oriental Medicine
http://www.aaaomonline.org/
English

The American Association of Acupuncture and Oriental Medicine (AAOM) aims to represent the professional Oriental medicine providers to ensure public confidence and to advocate the profession so that Oriental medicine providers will be given a status they deserve in the health care system. The Web site provides general information and conference news of the Association. Its contents are divided into "Member Services," "National Insurance Program," "American Acupuncturists," "Find an Acupuncturist," "Press Room," and "Annual Event."

A Guide to Chinese Medicine on the Internet

Asia's Medical System and Traditions
http://asianmedcom.site.securepod.com/home.htm
English

This Web site is sponsored by the Wellcome Trust Centre for the History of Medicine. It introduces the people and events of the Centre and courses supported by the Centre. It also introduces the key areas in history of Asian medicine and focuses on current research work in the field. Scholars associated with the Centre or previously funded by the Wellcome Trust continue to contribute to the study of Asian medicine.

Australian Traditional-Medicine Society
http://www.atms.com.au/
English

This is the Web site of the Australian Traditional-Medicine Society (ATMS), the largest professional association of complementary medicine practitioners in Australia. The organization, represents about 65 percent of the total complementary medicine profession, and is governed by the Executive Board of Directors with four main national committees. The Departments of Massage Therapy, Traditional Chinese Medicine, Homeopathy, Naturopathic Nutrition, Naturopathy and Western Herbal Medicine were established to address the specific needs of practitioners in these disciplines. The Web site publishes research essays on acupuncture, herbal medicine, nutrition, homeopathy and massage therapy, which can be read online. Also, it has other information like "Latest news," "Find a Practitioner," "Sites of Interest," "Code of Practice" and the society's own journal.

Biotechnology Research Institute: Traditional Chinese
Medicine Center, HKUST
http://www.ust.hk/%7Ebri/tcm.html
English

The Center is under the Biotechnology Research Institute of Hong Kong University of Science and Technology. It is divided into three groups: Bioassay and Drug Development Group, Safety and Standardization Group and Reformulation, and Pharmaceutics Group. The Center conducts a knowledge-based drug discovery effort. Biological assays are being utilized to screen TCM products and botanicals for therapeutically active compounds. The Web site introduces the Center.

California State Oriental Medicine Association
http://www.csomaonline.org/
English

The California State Oriental Medicine Association is a professional organization of licensed acupuncturists and Oriental medicine practitioners. Its objectives are to ensure the practice of Oriental medicine is provided in a caring and ethical manner so that the health of the general public will be enhanced. There is a basic introduction to Traditional Chinese Medicine on the Web site. The Web site provides news about the association and an introduction on the association's journal, *The California Journal of Oriental Medicine.*

Center for Arthritis and Traditional Chinese Medicine
http://nccam.nih.gov/training/centers/descriptions.htm#neuro1
English

This center (of Kernan Hospital and funded by NACCM) studies Traditional Chinese Medicine approaches—acupuncture and herbs—for the treatment of arthritis. Researchers conduct clinical trials of an eleven-herb Chinese formula (known as HLXL) for osteoarthritis of the knee; assess acupuncture's effect on inflammatory pain in an animal model; and study the efficacy of HLXL in an animal model of autoimmune arthritis.

Center for Chinese Herbal Therapy
http://nccam.nih.gov/training/centers/descriptions.htm#neuro1
English

The Center's (of Mount Sinai School of Medicine and funded by NACCM) researchers investigate a three-herb Chinese formula (known as ASHMI) as a therapy for allergic asthma. Studies of the herbal formula examine the mechanism of action in an animal model, characterize the herbs' active components, and investigate the formula's use in asthma patients.

Center for East-West Medicine, UCLA
http://www.cewm.med.ucla.edu/
English

The center offers educational program and conducts research on the integration of Chinese medicine with Western medicine.

Center of Excellence for the Neuroimaging of Acupuncture
    Effects on Human Brain Activity
http://www.nmr.mgh.harvard.edu/martinos/ctrFunding/
    acupuncturePPG.php
http://nccam.nih.gov/training/centers/descriptions.htm#neuro1
English

This Center (of Massachusetts General Hospital and funded by NACCM) aims to increase understanding of the neural basis for the effects of acupuncture through the use of functional magnetic resonance imaging. The Center will test the hypothesis that acupuncture generates a widespread response in the brain, and that the brain's limbic system plays a central role in this response. This organization explores the neural basis of *deqi,* a unique acupuncture sensation that is considered essential to clinical efficacy in traditional Chinese acupuncture.

China Academy of Chinese Medical Sciences
http://www.catcm.ac.cn/
Chinese (simplified) and English

China Academy of Chinese Medical Sciences is an important institute in the field of Chinese medicine, with its thirteen research institutes (such as The China Institute for History of Medicine and Medical Literatures, Institute of Acupuncture and Moxibustion, Institute of Information on Traditional Chinese Medicine, etc.), five hospitals (Xi Yuan Hospital is the most important one on Chinese medicine clinical research), four educational units, two museums, and two publishers. The Institute not only conducts research but also provides Chinese medical services in its hospitals, among which is a hospital of ophthalmology. The site offers news on Chinese medicine, including research, learning, and international academic activities. An English Web site is not available.

China Association of the Integrative Medicine
http://www.caim.org.cn/CN/index.html
Chinese (simplified)

The tenet of the association is to promote the integration of Western medicine and Traditional Chinese Medicine. The contents of its Web site include news, academic activities, journals, conference announcements, continuous education, conference agendas, international exchange, and an introduction to the association. It publishes the *Chinese Journal of Integrated Traditional and Western Medicine* and many other journals on the integration of Western and Chinese medicine. The association also holds academic conferences.

China Association of Chinese Medicine
http://218.241.72.18/webpage/zhzyyxh/index/
Chinese (simplified)

The China Association of Chinese Medicine (CACM) is a voluntary nonprofit organization formed by Traditional Chinese Medicine workers and legally registered TCM units throughout China. It is a national association affiliated with the China Association of Science and Technology, and also one of the institutions directly affiliated to the State Administration of Traditional Chinese Medicine. The China Association of Chinese Medicine was established in 1979. At present, CACM has 180,000 members, (of which 500 are overseas), and fifty-three special branches, and runs seventeen kinds of nationwide TCM periodicals. The contents of the Web site cover an introduction of the association, academic exchange, continuing education, international exchange, journals, technology development, awards, an introduction to experts, and book recommendations. It also publishes news on academic activities.

China International Exchange Center of Traditional Chinese
**   Medicine**
http://www.ciectcm.com/shtml/s-ciec-intro.htm
http://www.ciectcm.com/ehtml/e-index.htm
Chinese (simplified) and English

This is a nongovernmental, nonprofit institution directly supervised by the State Administration of Traditional Chinese Medicine, and specially engaged in the international nongovernmental exchange and cooperation on TCM. The Web site offers information on TCM hospitals, doctors, activities, products, training and publications, and it introduces its ten-year plan and cooperation partners worldwide.

China Medicine of Minorities
http://www.cmam.org.cn/
Chinese (simplified)

The organization aims to develop international academic exchange on medicine of minorities, to expound the discussion on academic topics in the field, the examination, evaluation and promotion of research achievements, to provide inquiry services for enterprises of medicine of minorities, to systematize the compilation and translation of literature on the topic, to develop the continue education of medicine of minorities and to recommend outstanding physicians of the field, in order to promote cultural exchange between different races.

Institute of Chinese Medicine, The Chinese University of Hong Kong
http://www.icm.cuhk.edu.hk/icm/
Chinese (traditional) and English

The Web site introduces the Institute of Chinese Medicine, its mission, organization, history, research, activities, and networks. The objective of the institute is to establish evidence-based Chinese medicine by performing the multiple functions of authentication, quality control, safety assurance, clinical trials, drug development, information center and public education, with a view to facilitating the cooperation between traditional and Western medicine.

Chinese Medical Sciences Data Center
http://test.cintcm.com/sjgx/
Chinese (simplified)

This site mainly builds and maintains TCM databases. The Web site offers news on TCM databases and introduces the contents of TCM databases. It offers links to demo databases.

Chinese Medicine Council of Hong Kong
http://www.cmchk.org.hk/
Chinese (traditional) and English

A statutory body established under the Chinese Medicine Ordinance, the Chinese Medicine Council of Hong Kong manages the practices and usages of Traditional Chinese Medicine in Hong Kong for the purposes of ensuring professional standards of Chinese medicine practice and protecting public health and consumer's rights. Its Web site provides Chinese medicine professionals, traders of Chinese medicines, and the public with the content of the Chinese Medicine Ordinance, which includes the composition and functions of the Chinese Medicine Council, framework of the regulatory system of Chinese medicine, and details of the regulatory measures. The Web site also provides an introduction of the council, the Chinese Medicine Ordinance, regulations of Chinese medicines, licensing of Chinese medicine traders, registration of patent Chinese medicines, the import and export control on Chinese medicines, the development of Chinese medicine in Hong Kong and reporting of adverse drug reactions. Users can also find news on Chinese Medicine in Hong Kong, documents of administrative policies, a list of toxic Chinese herbal medicines and the Chinese herbal medicines which are commonly used in Hong Kong.

Chinese Medicine Registration Board of Victoria
http://www.cmrb.vic.gov.au/
English

The Chinese Medicine Registration Board of Victoria was formed in December 2000 under the Chinese Medicine Registration Act 2000 with the intention to protect the public from fraudulent medical service. The Board registers Chinese herbal medicine practitioners, acupuncturists, and dispensers of Chinese herbs and conducts investigations into complaints about registrants' professional conduct or fitness to practice. The Web site publishes current issues and news, hearing and appeal decisions, registration, and information and instructions on how to make a complaint. It also provides newsletters and media releases. Users can download other relevant publications from the page.

Chinese Traditional Medicine Study
http://kanpougaku.com/kanpoukouza.html
Japanese

This organization studies Chinese medical formulae. Its Web site provides news about Traditional Chinese Medicine, a formulae search engine, explanations on terminologies, an introduction on dietetic therapy, and announcements of seminars.

College of TCM Practitioners and Acupuncturists of British Columbia
http://www.ctcma.bc.ca/index.asp
English

The College of TCM Practitioners and Acupuncturists of British Columbia (CTCMA) is an official professional licensing authority established in 1996 by the Government of British Columbia, Canada, to regulate the practice of Traditional Chinese Medicine and acupuncture in the Province. CTCMA is an expansion of the original College of Acupuncturists of British Columbia, which was created in 1996 by the government. The college is a self-regulatory body that operates under the auspices of the Provincial Government and through the Health Professions Act, the Traditional Chinese Medicine Practitioners and Acupuncturists Regulation and Bylaws. More than merely introducing the college, the Web site of the college provides additional information under these categories: "Introduction to TCM," "News & Events," "Regulations," "Meetings & Publications," and "Press Room." The Web site is also divided into three sections: "For Applicants," "For Registrants," and "For Public."

European Association of Traditional Chinese Medicine
http://www.eatcm.net/
English

The European Association of Traditional Chinese Medicine (EATCM) is an organization representing over 5,000 individuals in Europe working in the field of Chinese Medicine. Its aim is to spread information about Chinese Medicine for professionals and the public. The contents of its Web site include an introduction to the association, its members, status, news, and events.

European Institute of Oriental Medicine
http://www.eiom.de/
English and German

The European Institute of Oriental Medicine (EIOM), established in 2001, aims to provide education in traditional East Asian Medicine at undergraduate and postgraduate levels. It is a cooperative partner of the Arbeitsgemeinschaft für Klassische Akupunktur und Traditionelle Chinesische Medizin e. V, a European professional organization joining medical and nonmedical practitioners of Oriental medicine.

European Register of Organizations of TCM
http://www.euro-tcm.org/
English

The European Register of Organizations of TCM's (EURO-TCM) mission is the pursuit, preservation, and dissemination of knowledge and professionalism in Traditional Chinese Medicine. The Web site introduces the organizations and provides links relevant to Traditional Chinese Medicine. Also, downloadable sample issues of its journal, *The European Journal of Integrated Eastern and Western Medicine,* are available from the Web site.

**Foundation for Traditional Chinese Medicine: A Centre
  for Acupuncture Research**
http://www.ftcm.org.uk/
English

> The goal of the group is to bring the traditional Chinese system
> of acupuncture into the national health care system. The Web
> site provides an introduction on the foundation, its members,
> and current research projects (especially on acupunctural thera-
> pies treating back pain, depression, menorrhagia, chronic neck
> pain, and noncardiac chest pain; it also focuses on the Acupunc-
> ture Safety Projects, Chinese Herbs Safety Project, Neuroimag-
> ing of Acupuncture Project, and the Standards for Reporting
> Controlled Trials of Acupuncture (the STRICTA Project.) The
> research results can be downloaded from the Web site. Also,
> the annual reports from 2002 to 2005 and essays published by
> the members are available.

Functional Bowel Disorders in Chinese Medicine
http://nccam.nih.gov/training/centers/descriptions.htm#neuro1
English

> This center (of Kernan Hospital and funded by NACCM) con-
> ducts multidisciplinary research on Traditional Chinese Medi-
> cine (TCM) practices–acupuncture and herbs—for the treatment
> of irritable bowel syndrome (IBS). Researchers study effects of
> acupuncture and a TCM herbal preparation in an animal model
> of IBS, and conduct a preliminary study of the herbal prepara-
> tion with IBS patients (Web site, NCCAM).

Hong Kong Association of Traditional Chinese Medicine
http://www.chinesemedicinehka.com/
Chinese (traditional)

> The Web site gives an introduction on the association, and it
> also introduces common Traditional Chinese Medicine and
> Chinese dietotherapy. It has a database that lists registered Chi-

nese medical physicians in Hong Kong. Users can search for registered physicians by locations.

Hong Kong Jockey Club Institute of Chinese Medicine Ltd
http://www.hkjcicm.org
Chinese (simplified and traditional), English

This is an organization under the auspices of the Hong Kong Jockey Club. It supports the development of Traditional Chinese Medicine in Hong Kong and subsidizes relevant research projects. Its mission is to develop Chinese medicine as a high value-added industry for Hong Kong through promotion and coordination of related activities and strategic support for scientific and evidence-based development programs. It has been participating in the strategy formulation for TCM development in Hong Kong, supporting TCM-related scientific research, coordinating and managing R&D programs and promotion of commercialization of R&D results, participating in the enhancement of safety, quality, and efficacy and the promotion of Good Agricultural Practice, Good Manufacturing Practice, Good Laboratory Practice and Good Clinical Practice, and gathering information in Hong Kong, Mainland China, and overseas relating to R&D activities. Its Web site includes "What's New," "About HKJCICM," "Our Portfolio," "Business Development," "Funding," "Newsletter," and "Major Events."

Institute for Traditional Medicine
http://www.itmonline.org/
English

The Institute for Traditional Medicine (ITM) and Preventive Health Care, Inc. is a nonprofit organization. ITM was founded by and is directed by Subhuti Dharmananda, PhD. The institute operates two clinical facilities, the Immune Enhancement Project and the An Hao Natural Health Care Clinic. It provides research essays on Traditional Chinese Medicine written by Subhuti Dharmananda online for free (under the section of Start

Group). The institute provides herbal formulations by practitioners who study ITM's literature. ITM also contributes to the preservation of traditional medicine. Nevertheless, ITM is not a school and does not offer courses, certifications, or diplomas, and it does not conduct clinical or laboratory research.

Institute of Information on Traditional Chinese Medicine
http://www.cintcm.ac.cn/
Chinese (simplified)

This is a very important institute for collecting, disseminating, and analyzing information on TCM, both locally and internationally. The institute develops many useful and crucial databases about Chinese medicine, and publishes journals. The site also has a section of "Encyclopedia for Chinese medicine," "Chinese medicine in U.S and Europe market" and "Digital Information and Modernization of Chinese medicine."

International Association for the Study of Traditional Asian
   Medicine
http://www.iastam.org/
English

The International Association for the Study of Traditional Asian Medicine is an international organization that aims to embrace both academics and practitioners in the field of Asian medicine by providing a platform for these groups to express their views and for the exchange of knowledge. Its Web site presents the history and news announcements of the association. It also introduces its newsletter and journal, *Asian Medicine*. Under the column "services," users can download "online exhibitions" on Traditional Chinese Medicine.

**International Center of Traditional Chinese Medicine
  for Cancer
http://nccam.nih.gov/news/2005/101405.htm
English**

> The International Center of Traditional Chinese Medicine for Cancer (of M.D. Anderson Cancer Center, Houston and funded by NACCM) conducts preclinical and clinical studies of Traditional Chinese Medicine approaches—herbs, acupuncture, and Qigong—for treating cancer and its symptoms, as well as treatment-related side effects.

**International Chinese Medicine Society
http://www.akupunktur.ch/start.html
English and German**

> Based in Germany, the Web site introduces Traditional Chinese Medicine, including acupuncture, herbal medicine, Qigong and yin-yang. It has recommendations on Traditional Chinese Medicine books written in German.

**International Society for Chinese Medicine
http://www.iscm.org.mo/
Chinese (traditional) and English**

> The International Society for Chinese Medicine, based in Macau, publishes *Chinese Medicine*. The Web site introduces details of the society, including its publications, conferences, and academic exchange. The society aims to unite international experts to disseminate Chinese medicine research through international, interdisciplinary, and interinstitutional collaborations for the modernization and internationalization of Chinese medicine. It advocates the pursuit of evidence-based approaches to clinical and laboratory research in Chinese medicine among academic and research institutions worldwide.

International Society of Oriental Medicine
http://www.isom.or.kr/
English and Korean

The International Society of Oriental Medicine was founded in
1976 with the intention to promote Oriental medicine and medicine of all humanity regardless of the indigenous or national
medicine limits. It holds international congress and seminars,
carries out research, exchange, and development of Oriental
medicine. It also establishes an information network through
exchange of information. Its content includes congress, document, community, and ISOM news.

Modernized Chinese Medicine International Association
http://www.mcmia.org/
Chinese (simplified and traditional) and English

This organization is located in Hong Kong. Its aim is to provide
the latest information and commercial opportunities in Chinese
medicine to its global membership, the association holds conferences, seminars, exhibitions, training courses, regular meetings, and field trips. It also contributes to the research, education
and worldwide promotion of Chinese medicine. Furthermore,
MCMIA supports Hong Kong government's plan to establish
Hong Kong as an international center for Chinese medicine and
will compile and forward its members' views and opinions on
this issue to the authority. Its Web site introduces the association and provides news about Traditional Chinese Medicine in
Hong Kong.

NESA Acupuncture Research Collaborative
http://nccam.nih.gov/training/centers/descriptions.htm
  #acupuncture
English

This Developmental Center for Research (of New England
School of Acupuncture and funded by NACCM) brings togeth-

er leaders from the Oriental medicine (OM) and conventional medicine communities to critically evaluate the efficacy and safety of acupuncture, and to develop sound methodologies for acupuncture research. The center builds upon ongoing collaborations between the NESA and two other HMS-affiliated institutions, and the Dana Farber Cancer Institute and Children's Hospital Boston. The center supports three exploratory studies, including one that assesses the reliability of a method for reaching traditional OM diagnoses in the context of clinical trials. This study also explores issues related to the individualization of acupuncture treatments in the context of clinical trials, appropriate controls for acupuncture clinical trials, and the development of outcome measures consistent with the philosophy of traditional OM. Other studies assess the benefits of acupuncture as an adjunct therapy in the treatment of chronic pain in young women with endometriosis, and in the treatment of women with ovarian cancer who are receiving chemotherapy. Academic and administrative mentoring programs are an integral part of this center's mission. An important goal of the center will be to enable NESA to play the lead role in the future submission to NIH of competitive applications that build upon these exploratory studies.

Pan European Federation of TCM Societies
http://www.pefots.com/
English

The Pan European Federation of TCM Societies (PEFOTS) aims to develop TCM education, the TCM profession, and research. It contributes to TCM education by holding a yearly academic conference with seminars focused on various themes to enhance the quality of TCM practice. The contents of its Web site include news, statutes, associations, boards, and working commissions.

Professional Committee of Traditional Chinese Medicine
http://www.zyyw.com/zhishudanwei.htm
Chinese (simplified)

The site introduces the committee and its working projects. One of the projects is to build a "City of Chinese Medical Science" in Beijing. The laws of Chinese medicine and related documents are also found on the Web site.

Shanghai Chinese Medical Document House
http://www.zywxg.com/
Chinese (simplified)

Its work is to provide Chinese medicine information and publish journals such as *Zhong yi wen xian za zhi* (Journal of Chinese medical documents) and *Shang hai zhong yi you qing bao* (Friendly journal for Shanghai Chinese physicians). In addition, it also provides clinical service. TCM Search Center (http://www.zywxg.com/cxjs .htm) and *Zhong yi yao ke ji fu wu zhong xin* (Chinese Medical Technology Service Center http://www.zywxg.com/zykyfwzx.htm) are the subunits of the house. The former helps clients search Chinese medical documents, and the latter allows clients to monitor research progress.

State Administration of Traditional Chinese Medicine
   of the People's Republic of China
http://www.satcm.gov.cn/
Chinese (simplified)

It is the official institute that manages TCM affairs in China, including supervision and administration. There are eight units under its supervision, such as China Academy of Chinese Medical Sciences. The site offers news and laws about Chinese medicine, and links to academic bodies and universities of TCM.

The Accreditation Commission for Acupuncture and Oriental Medicine
http://www.acaom.org/
English

The Accreditation Commission for Acupuncture and Oriental Medicine accredits Master's level programs in Oriental medicine, especially acupuncture and herbal therapie; recognized by the U.S. Department of Education.

The Association of Traditional Chinese Medicine U.K
http://cmauk.org/cmauk/Atcmuk.html (page not found, try
http://www.atcm.co.uk)
English

The Association of Traditional Chinese Medicine (UK) Limited, founded in 1994, aims to promote proper professional qualifications and high standards of medical services among Traditional Chinese Medicine practitioners.

The Australian Acupuncture and Chinese Medicine Association Ltd.
http://www.acupuncture.org.au/
English

The Australian Acupuncture and Chinese Medicine Association Ltd. is a national professional association of acupuncture and Traditional Chinese Medicine practitioners. Its objective is to maintain high standards of education and practice. Not only does the Web site introduce the organization, it provides information on health services, finding a practitioner, studying TCM, and other relevant news. The organization publishes a newsletter, *Jing-Luo,* which together with the *Australian Journal of Acupuncture and Chinese Medicine* are both downloadable.

The Chinese Medical Physician Qualification Center
http://www.tcmtest.com.cn/
Chinese (simplified)

The center is under the State Administration of Traditional Chinese Medicine. It is responsible for the qualification examination for doctors of Chinese medicine. The site offers information of the examinations.

The Institute of Basic Medicine of TCM, Academy of Chinese Medical Sciences
http://www.ibmtcm.ac.cn/
Chinese (simplified)

The Web site introduces the organization, research, and publications of the institute. There are many articles related to the basics of TCM on the Web. The institute also publishes the *Chinese Journal of Basic Medicine of Traditional Chinese Medicine.*

The Japan Kampo Medicine Association
http://www.nihonkanpoukyokai.com/
Japanese

The Web site introduces the structure and history of the association and posts announcements for its conferences.

The Japan Society for Oriental Medicine
http://www.jsom.or.jp/html/index.htm
English and Japanese

The society aims to contribute to the development of scientific culture in Oriental medicine by holding research presentations, communicating the promotion concerning Oriental medicine, and contributing to the progress and dissemination of Oriental medicine. The Japan Society for Oriental Medicine issues the journal *Kampo Medicine* and other publications. It also operates the medical specialist certification program of JSOM. The Web site provides news of the society, and it publishes the index of *Kampo Medicine*. It has a database of Chinese physicians in Japan, which users can search by location. Also, information of seminars can be found. The Japanese version contains more information.

The National Union of Chinese Medical Doctors' Association R.O.C
http://www.uncma.org.tw/
Chinese (traditional)

It introduces the association and its history and development. It also provides elementary knowledge of traditional Chinese health care. Users can also read the "Chinese Health Care Handbook" published by the association, and abstracts of essays published in *Taiwan Journal of Chinese Medicine.*

The Acupuncture and Oriental Medicine Association of New Mexico
http://www.omanm.org/
English

The Acupuncture and Oriental Medicine Association of New Mexico is a nonprofit, professional organization that promotes the practice of acupuncture and Oriental medicine. It also upholds excellence in the professional and ethical standards of its members. Its Web site introduces the association and its members. It also publishes online articles on Traditional Chinese Medicine and acupuncture.

The Society of Clinical Traditional Chinese Medicine in Japan
http://www.mmjp.or.jp/kampo-ikai/
Japanese

More than providing information of the society and its members, the Web site introduces basic knowledge of Traditional Chinese Medicine.

The Society of Traditional Chinese Medicine of Jilin Province
http://www.sinew.com.cn/zhong/index.htm
Chinese (simplified)

> The Web site presents the society, its activities, members, and famous Chinese physicians. It also introduces knowledge of Traditional Chinese Medicine.

TCM meetings in Europe: The site of the largest annual
European TCM conference (Rothenburg)
http://www.tcm-kongress.de/
English and German (with an introduction available in French,
simplified Chinese, Dutch, Spanish, Hebrew and Swedish)

> The TCM conference held annually by Arbeitsgemeinschaft für Klassische Akupunktur und TCM e. V. is a not-for-profit event that aims to offer knowledge related to Chinese medicine and to demonstrate its variety throughout history. It discusses not only the classical therapies of acupuncture, *Materia Medica,* Tuina, Qigong, etc., but also subjects like Feng Shui. It presents different schools of thought without any dogmatism. The Web site introduces the conference's history, information, program, speakers, literature, and video/audio recording.

Traditional Chinese Medicine Association & Alumni
http://www.tcmaa.org
English

> Traditional Chinese Medicine Association & Alumni (TC-MAA), headquartered in New York City, is the largest professional organization of Traditional Chinese Medicine (TCM) on the East Coast of the United States. It organizes conferences and symposiums in Traditional Chinese Medicine and publishes the *American Journal of Traditional Chinese Medicine* and *Inner Vision,* an official news letter of TCMAA. The Web site provides TCMAA conferences, news, TCM Union Issues,

newsletters, and many other links related to Traditional Chinese Medicine.

Traditional Chinese Medicine World Foundation
http://www.tcmworld.org/
English

The Traditional Chinese Medicine World Foundation is a non-profit organization dedicated to promoting classical Traditional Chinese Medicine and natural healing. Its Web site includes an introduction to acupuncture, tui na, and the fundamentals of Traditional Chinese Medicine. *Harmony,* the newsletter published by this organization, can also be downloaded for free.

Traditional Clinical Chinese Medicine Association
http://www.sino-medicine.com.tw/~cctcma/index-e-1.htm
Chinese (traditional)

The purpose of the association is for the research and education of basic and clinical Traditional Chinese Medicine. Its Web site provides news, and users can read its *Journal of China Clinical Traditional Medicine* online for free.

World Federation of Chinese Medicine Societies
http://www.wfcms.org/
Chinese (simplified)

The Web site provides news of the federation and of the field of Traditional Chinese Medicine. It also introduces Chinese medicinal materials. Links to TCM organizations are also available.

ACUPUNCTURE

Acupuncture Association of Washington
http://www.waoma.org/
English

The founders of the Acupuncture Association of Washington were integral in helping to establish Oriental medicine as a legal practice in Washington State. The Web site introduces Traditional Chinese Medicine and acupuncture.

Acupuncture and Oriental Medicine Association of Minnesota
http://www.aomam.org/
English

The Acupuncture and Oriental Medicine Association of Minnesota (AOMAM) is an organization that supports the acupuncture and Oriental medicine profession in the state of Minnesota. Its objective is to advance the profession of acupuncture and Oriental medicine within the state of Minnesota by supporting its members through continuing education, legislative activities, and as a link to national developments and research within our profession. Its Web site provides news and introduces members of the association, and it also gives a brief introduction on acupuncture, Traditional Chinese Medicine and its history. Most of the content of the Web site is still under construction.

Acupuncture and Oriental Medicine National Coalition
http://www.aomnc.com/
English

The Web site introduces the Acupuncture and Oriental Medicine National Coalition, an organization that aims to advance acupuncture and Oriental medicine by promoting "qualified licensees" and its full acceptance in both the private and governmental health care arena.

Acupuncture Sans Frontiers
http://perso.wanadoo.fr/acusf/
English, French, Italian, and Spanish

The Acupuncture Sans Frontiers, established in 1992 in France, is a nonprofit independent organization. It aims to promote development of a greater autonomy of public health treatment in the third world countries by using therapeutic alternatives. The Web site introduces the Frontier and its administration.

Acupuncture Society of New York
http://www.asny.org/
English

The Acupuncture Society of New York, established in 1990, aims to promote the growth of the acupuncture profession in the New York State. It serves the public through lectures, publications, referral service, and by providing information on its Web site. It also serves the profession though legislative work, national conferences and organizations, continuing education, and publications. Its Web site gives an introduction on the society. It also introduces acupuncture and posts relevant research essays. The society publishes *Meridian Times,* of which six articles from past issues are available online. The site has columns like "discussion groups" and "practice issues"; the former is for discussion on Traditional Chinese Medicine, and the latter deals with acupuncture, related insurance issues, and practice management.

American Academy of Medical Acupuncture
http://www.medicalacupuncture.org/aama_marf/aama.html
English

The American Academy of Medical Acupuncture aims to promote the integration of concepts from traditional and modern forms of acupuncture with Western medical training. The Academy publishes *Medical Acupuncture: A Journal for Physi-*

cians by Physicians. The Web site mainly provides news of the Academy.

British Acupuncture Accreditation Board
http://www.acupuncture.org.uk/content/baab/baab.html
English

The purpose of the Board is to accredit institutions who offer acupunctural courses. The standards of accreditation is based on the Guidelines for Acupuncture Education established by the Board and the British Acupuncture Council. The Web site provides a downloadable BAAB Annual Report 2004 and Accreditation Handbook Online August 2005.

Canadian Association of Acupuncture and Traditional Chinese Medicine
http://www.caatcm.com/
Chinese (traditional) and English

The Web site introduces the structure of the association, its goals, its members, and related news.

Canadian Chinese Medicine and Acupuncture Association
http://www.cmaac.ca
English

The aims of the association are to solidify practitioners of Oriental and Western medicine, set up standards of education and training, lobby the government for regulation of Chinese medicine and acupuncture. The Web site is an introduction to the association. It also publishes a progress report and other news on Traditional Chinese Medicine in Canada.

Chinese Medical Association of Acupuncture
http://www.cmaa.org.tw/
Chinese (traditional)

This organization was established for the study and development of acupuncture, to strengthen the exchange between Chinese and Western medicine, within and outside of China, in order to enhance acupunctural medicine. The Web site introduces the association, news of its academic conferences, tables of contents, and abstracts of its publication *Journal of Chinese Medical Association of Acupuncture* and other news.

Chinese Association of Acupuncture and Moxibustion
http://www.caam.cn/
Chinese (simplified)

The Chinese Association of Acupuncture and Moxibustion deals with the development of acupunctural academic exchange within and outside of China, technological inquiries and services, scientific investigation, clinical acupuncture, continue education, achievement promotion, popularization of science, etc. The association has fifteen subsocieties and working groups.

The World Federation of Acupuncture-Moxibustion Societies
http://www.wfas.com.cn/
Chinese (simplified)

The group serves to organize worldwide acupunctural academic conferences and meetings, to propagate and promote acupunctural science, to fight for legal status of acupuncture in every nation, to develop acupunctural education and to publish the acupunctural academic journal, *World Acupuncture Magazine*. The Web site has very detailed information on the society and its member societies. If readers would like to know acupuncture organizations in the world, the site has a full list.

Council of Colleges of Acupuncture and Oriental Medicine
http://www.ccaom.org/
English

The mission of the Council of Colleges of Acupuncture and Oriental Medicine (CCAOM) aims to advance acupuncture and Oriental medicine by promoting education within the field. This Web site introduces the council's structure and its member schools. The newsletter of the council is available online.

European Acupuncture Association
http://www.aea-org.com/
English and French

The Web site introduces the history of the association, its structure, and its goals. It also posts latest news, information on public health in E.U. publications by E.U. and other acupuncture Web site and articles.

Federation of Acupuncture and Oriental Medicine Regulatory Agencies
http://www.faomra.com/
English

Created in 1999, the Federation of Acupuncture and Oriental Medicine Regulatory Agencies helps to regulate the practice of Oriental medicine as health care, develops suggestions for licensing procedures, trains students, and communicates information to the public at large. Agencies are encouraged to become members, and an annual meeting is held. The Web site introduces the federation and its members.

Illinois Association of Acupuncture & Oriental Medicine
http://www.ilaaom.org/
English

The Illinois Association of Acupuncture & Oriental Medicine is a professional organization representing licensed acupuncturists and students in Illinois. The Web site provides an introduction to Traditional Chinese Medicine, news of the association and legislative information. Visitors can read articles and book reviews regarding Traditional Chinese Medicine on this Web site.

Institute of Acupuncture and Moxibustion, China Academy of Chinese Medical Sciences
http://iam.acutimes.com/
Chinese (simplified) and English

This is the most important acupuncture research institute in China. The purpose of the institute is to engage well-rounded acupuncture research, including creating acupuncture databases, publishing academic journals, conducting research, exploiting acupuncture software, maintaining museums, etc. The institute has seven research centers: Center for Basic Theories of Acupuncture, Center for Acupuncture and Molecular Biology, Center for Meridians Research, Center for Clinical Evaluation and Standardization of Acupuncture, etc. The site introduces its organization, research results, postgraduate education, academic exchange and journals *(Chinese Acupuncture and Moxibustion, Acupuncture Research,* and *World Journal of Acupuncture and Moxibustion).* English Web site is not available.

International Council of Medical Acupuncture and Related Techniques
http://www.icmart.org/
English

The council is an organization that unites over eighty medical acupuncture societies and 3,000 practitioners of acupuncture around the world. The Web site introduces the council, which supports academic conferences on acupuncture. On the Web site visitors can find information regarding academic acupuncture conferences held and sponsored by the council, abstracts of essays, and an introduction to research in acupuncture.

International Academy of Medical Acupuncture
http://www.iama.edu/
English

The Academy is dedicated to teaching both the ancient as well as contemporary principles of acupuncture. The Web site gives an introduction to acupuncture and research articles on acupuncture written by John A. Amaro. It also provides articles, electro/meridian imaging, and other great resources.

Korean Acupuncture and Moxibustion Society
http://www.acumoxa.or.kr/eng/
English and Korean

The Korean Acupuncture and Moxibustion Society was established in 1973 as a section of the Korean Oriental Medical society. Its mission is to contribute to the development of acupuncture and moxibustion and promotion of people's health and has led various academic activities. The Web site introduces the society, information regarding its research, educational activities, and conferences.

Michigan Medical Acupuncture Association
http://www.michiganmedicalacupuncture.org/
English

This association of acupuncturists is the largest in Michigan and seeks to reach out to the public to communicate about the safety and effectiveness of acupuncture. Although this organization is particular to one U.S. state, the Web site provides additional information about techniques, standards of practice, and certification. An extensive list of Web resources on acupuncture is also presented. The site posts research essays on acupuncture and pictures showing acupuncture techniques.

National Acupuncture and Oriental Medicine Alliance
http://acuall.org/
English

> The NAOMA is a not-for-profit group that seeks to communicate to the public about Oriental medicine as well as to effect policy changes at the state and national level. This organization has a referral service for people interested in receiving acupuncture, it is working to pass new legislation about acupuncture in numerous states, lobbies for more visibility for acupuncture and Oriental medicine in current health care practices, and seeks to get Oriental medicine covered more fully by health insurance companies. The Web site for NAOMA also includes links for general information on acupuncture and Oriental medicine, including a list of contact information for national organizations. The AOM Alliance maintains this Web site for consumers, practitioners, students, and everyone who is interested in the field. The organization is committed to improving public health through acupuncture and Oriental medicine. The Web site provides free newsletters, a forum, and it introduces publications on Chinese medicine publications and Chinese medical schools.

National Acupuncture Detoxification Association
http://www.acudetox.com/
English

> The association is an educational corporation which conducts education and training of the specific auricular (ear) acupuncture. Its goals are to make acupunctural treatment popular and to integrate acupuncture and other curing methods.

**National Certification Commission for Acupuncture
   and Oriental Medicine**
http://www.nccaom.org/
English

> Established in 1982, the purpose of the commission is to set up
> and promote recognized safety standards of using acupuncture
> and Oriental medicine. It provides certification programs. The
> Web site provides relevant information for practitioners, diplo-
> mats, and applicants, respectively.

New Zealand Register of Acupuncturists
http://www.acupuncture.org.nz/
English

> The New Zealand Register of Acupuncturists was incorporated
> as a society in 1977 to promote Traditional Chinese Medicine.
> On the Web site, one can find lists of registered acupuncturists
> in acupuncture colleges in New Zealand. The Web site also in-
> troduces acupuncture therapies.

Society for Acupuncture Research
http://www.acupunctureresearch.org/
English

> The Society for Acupuncture Research is a nonprofit organiza-
> tion that aims to promote scientific research in the clinical effi-
> cacy, physiological mechanisms, patterns of use, and theoretical
> foundations of acupuncture, herbal therapy, and other modali-
> ties of Oriental medicine. *The Journal of Alternative and Com-
> plementary Medicine* is the official journal of the society.

Society of Auricular Acupuncturists
http://www.auricularacupuncture.org.uk/
English

> The Web site introduces the society and auricular acupuncture.
> It has information on auricular acupuncture courses.

The American Board of Medical Acupuncture
http://www.dabma.org/index.asp
English

> In 2000, the American Board of Medical Acupuncture (ABMA) was created as a part of the American Academy of Medical Acupuncture (AAMA). The Board's goal is to develop standards of practice and certify practitioners as acupuncture specialists by holding exams, qualifying students, certifying physicians, and promoting the use of acupuncture in health care. The Web site details the process of board certification, which involves educational experience, an examination, and practical experience as well. Interested parties can use the Web site to apply to be a board-certified medical acupuncture specialist, and the Web site maintains a list of certified practitioners. The contents of the Web site include "board certification process," "exam validation process," "recommended readings for the exam," "ABMA Board of Trustees," and "board certified physicians."

The British Acupuncture Council
http://www.acupuncture.org.uk/
English

> The British Acupuncture Council (BAcC) represents professional acupuncturists in the United Kingdom and encourages its members to practice a recognized and traditional style of diagnosis and treatment therapy. It provides downloadable research documents on acupuncture and a British practitioner search. The British Acupuncture Council is the organization that publishes the journal, *The European Journal of Oriental Medicine*.

The British Medical Acupuncture Society
http://www.medical-acupuncture.co.uk/
English

The British Medical Acupuncture Society (BMAS) is a registered charity established to encourage the use and scientific understanding of acupuncture within medicine for the public benefit. The Web site is categorized into "News and Forum" for members, "Meeting and Courses," "Software Reviewers," "Hot Topics in Acupuncture" and "Acupuncture Supplies" for professionals, and "Information for Patients," "London Teaching Clinic" and "Find a Practitioner" for patients. It provides news and basic knowledge of acupuncture. The homepage of the British Medical Acupuncture Society includes a free newsletter and subscription information for paper and electronic versions for its journal, *Acupuncture in Medicine.*

The Japan Society of Acupuncture and Moxibustion
http://www.jsam.jp/
English and Japanese

The Web site introduces the society, its news, and two academic journals, *Journal of JSAM* and *Japanese Acupuncture and Moxibustion* (online journal). Also, a search engine is available for searching periodicals. Information on recent research and development of history of acupuncture in Japan can be found on the page.

The Japanese Acupuncturist Society
http://www.zensin.or.jp/
Japanese

The Web site introduces the society, its history, and member listing. It also has links to its branches in each Japanese prefecture.

**The Association of Acupuncture and Moxibustion-Clinical
  Society**
http://www.zgzjxh.cn/
Chinese (simplified)

> The Clinical Society is a subsociety of The Association of Acupuncture and Moxibustion. The Web site introduces its organization, publications, activities, and training courses. The site also provides news and academic articles on the Web.

HERBAL

American Botanical Council
http://www.herbalgram.org/
English

> Established in 1988, the American Botanical Council is a nonprofit international organization providing education using science-based and traditional information to promote the responsible use of herbal medicine. The Web site provides online resources on herbal information, including news and educational resources. The council publishes *HerbalGram: The Journal of the American Botanical Council,* and free selected articles and free sample issues are available on the Web site. Moreover, there is "HerbClip" that provides relevant reviews, "Healthy Ingredients" that introduces plants and related materials used in dietary supplements and natural cosmetics, and "HerbMedPro," which is an herbal database that provides hyperlinked access to the scientific data underlying the use of herbs for health. However, these services are limited to member use.

British Herbal Medicine Association
http://www.escop.com/bhma/bhma/frame.htm
English

> Found in 1964, the association aims to promote the science and
> practice of herbal medicine and to use herbal remedies safety.
> It also considers that herbal medicine has its own value and
> should be a choice for the patients. Latest documents related
> to herbal medicine are collected under the column "Essential
> Reading."

Canadian Institute of Chinese Medicinal Research
http://www.bepress.com/jcim/cicmr.html
English

> The institute promotes the safe use of Chinese medicine in Can-
> ada. It considers that achieving this mission should be based on
> conducting research, training the practitioners, and educating
> the users of Chinese medicine.

Center for International Ethnomedicinal Education
   and Research
http://www.cieer.org/
English

> CIEER was founded in 1998 as a nonprofit organization that
> deals with the dissemination of traditional botanical knowl-
> edge. This group seeks to educate the public about the medici-
> nal uses of plants as well as to preserve traditional approaches
> to botanical medicines in a variety of languages. The Web site
> for CIEER offers a wealth of information, from colleges and
> universities that offer programs in ethnobotany to conferences
> that deal with botanical medicine. There is a discussion forum
> and a Listserv, both of which are free to join. The links to proj-
> ects and education provide additional information on how stu-
> dents can get involved in ethnobotany, and the resource direc-
> tory has collected links to numerous Web sites, bibliographies,

and professional societies. The Web site lists and posts online the research achievements and publications of the center. It also provides information about courses for ethnomedicine.

European Herbal and Traditional Medicine Practitioners Association
http://www.ehpa.eu/index.html
English

The Association aims to foster unity within the herbal profession, to promote professional herbal treatment, and to raise standards of training and practice within the profession. It advocates the legalization of professional herbal practice throughout the EU as a speciality in its own right. The Web site also introduces Chinese herbal medicine. The association's newsletter is also available. The Web site includes "Statutory regulation," "Medicine Legislation," and "Standards."

European Society for Classical Natural Medicine
http://www.escnm.de/
English, German, and Spanish (French section is currently unavailable)

This society was founded in order to promote the use of what they call "classical natural medicine," which includes practices such as massage therapy, nutrition, medicinal plant use, heliotherapy, and fasting. The society seeks to gather information about practices that have been rigorously tested scientifically. The Web site is multilingual, and there are working groups on such topics as immunology, fasting, and quality assurance. The society plans to hold annual meetings, to be active in designing curricula for students, and to inform the public about classical natural medicine. The Web site introduces classical natural medicine and explores further characteristics.

European Society of Ethnopharmacology
http://ethnopharma.free.fr/
English

In 1990, the European Society of Ethnopharmacology was founded as an organization whose members are interested in pharmacopoeias. Members include specialists from a wide range of disciplines, such as medical doctors, anthropologists, and historians; it publishes a bulletin twice a year. The society is active in creating and participating in research projects and in holding international conferences. The Web site is easily accessible, with an excellent layout that presents information, its officers, publications, and conferences. An additional page offers contact information and links to a variety of professional organizations and other Internet resources. The Web site describes the details of the society and its related news. It introduces *Ethnopharmacologia,* along with the index of each issue, other publications by members, and proceedings of congresses.

Herb Research Foundation
http://herbs.org/index.html#about
English

The Herb Research Foundation provides information on the health benefits and safety of herbs. The Web site posts headlines and press releases of herbal research. It has sections like "Sustainable Development," and "Services and Resources," which provide an introduction to research achievements and other relevant links.

Institute of Medicinal Plant Development
http://www.implad.ac.cn/
Chinese (simplified) and English

In 1983, the Institute of Medicinal Plant Development was created in Beijing, China, and today has locations in several other Chinese provinces as well. The goal of IMPLAD is to preserve knowledge about plant use in Traditional Chinese Medicine and to utilize modern technology to further develop this practice. Some of the fields that the 680 researchers are interested in include pharmacology, toxicology, and chemistry. IMPLAD has participated in both national and international projects dealing with medicinal plants. The Institute's Web site, available in both Chinese and English, provides information about research departments and branches, as well as biographies and photographs of numerous professors and experts on staff. The site discusses the institute in details and offers news about medicinal plants.

International Society of Ethnopharmacology
http://www.ethnopharmacology.org/
English

The society promotes ethnopharmacology as a scientific research discipline, and its past and upcoming congresses and conferences. The society publishes *Journal of Ethnopharmacology: An Interdisciplinary Journal Devoted to Indigenous Drugs*. The newsletter is downloadable.

National Herbalist Association of Australia
http://www.nhaa.org.au/index.htm
English

The National Herbalist Association of Australia is the oldest natural therapies association in Australia. Its aims are to promote, protect, and encourage the study, practice, and knowledge of medical herbalism, to disseminate knowledge, seminars, and publications, and to encourage the highest ideals of professional and ethical standards. The contents of its Web site relate to Traditional Chinese Medicine. The Web site introduces the organization, its members, and herbal medicine. The organization publishes a free newsletter and *Australian Journal of Medical Herbalism*.

Sichuan Institute of Chinese Materia Medica
http://www.sicmm.com.cn/
Chinese (simplified) and English

In 1930, the Sichuan Institute of Chinese Materia Medica was founded in Nanjing, China, although it is currently housed in Cheng Du. This institute has numerous departments whose research and development assist in understanding and furthering the practice of Traditional Chinese Medicine. The institute boasts a staff of over 160 people, and their work has resulted in several patents and new drugs. The Web site introduces the institute and collects news on Chinese *Materia Medica* and the modernization of Chinese medicine. The English version only briefly introduces the institute and does not have any information on Chinese *Materia Medica*.

Society for Medicinal Plant Research
http://www.ga-online.org/index.html
English and German

The Society for Medicinal Plant Research was founded in Germany in 1953 as an organization dedicated to the study of medicinal plants. Its current goal reflects its original purpose and includes a commitment to scientific analysis and information dissemination. In addition to organizing scientific meetings and providing financial support for research, the society publishes a journal called *Planta Medica: Natural Products and Medicinal Plant Research*. The cost of membership in the society is low, and membership brings with it abstracts from the annual meeting and information on upcoming lectures and conferences.

Tang Center for Herbal Medicine Research
http://tangcenter.uchicago.edu/
English

The Tang Center, based at the University of Chicago, was founded in 2000 with the goal of using the scientific method to understand both the efficacy of herbs in curing disease as well as the side effects and toxicity of herbal remedies. The center also produces herbal formulations, offers course instruction to students, and informs consumers of the pros and cons of herbal supplement use. Recent research by scholars includes the "Textbook of Complementary and Alternative Medicine" by Chun-Su Yuan. The Web site provides information on numerous research projects and publications, as well as a page listing external sites that deal with herbal resources. The Web site introduces the Center and its research projects with the latest achievements. The Center provides herbal resources, and it publishes *American Journal of Chinese Medicine.*

The Chinese Medicinal Plants Authentication Centre
http://www.rbgkew.org.uk/scihort/ecbot/ecbot-cmpac.html
English

Housed at the Royal Botanical Gardens at Kew in London, England, is the Chinese Medicinal Plants Authentication Centre (CMPAC). It is a nonprofit center for scientific understanding of Chinese herbs, and its goals are to develop quality assurance guidelines, to train researchers and practitioners of Chinese herbal medicine, and to conserve the medicinal plants currently known. Medicinal preparations can be sent to CMPAC, where their components will be analyzed with a battery of scientific tests. The Centre's Web site includes information about cost of testing samples, recently published research, and contact information.

The Herb Society of America
http://www.herbsociety.org
English

The Web site introduces the details of the Herb Society of America, which is dedicated to promoting the knowledge and use of herbs.

The Register of Chinese Herbal Medicine
http://www.rchm.co.uk/
English

The Register of Chinese Herbal Medicine is a clearinghouse for information on a variety of topics related to the understanding and practice of herbal medicine. Created in 1987 as a regulatory agency of Chinese herbal medicine in the United Kingdom, the RCHM provides information on practitioners and instructors of Chinese herbal medicine, deals with regulation and quality of herbs, and provides information to the public and to the media on the safety and efficacy of herbal medicines. The Web site for the RCHM includes a wealth of information about herbal medicine, including a section on FAQs, schools that train practitioners, as well as a case history database that is free for any registered user. Membership is also available, the price of which includes a subscription to the semi-annual journal of the RCHM. It also introduces Traditional Chinese Medicine and Chinese medical therapy. It has an introduction to the Bristol Chinese Herb Garden and other essays on Chinese medical research.

QIGONG AND RELATED FIELDS

American Massage Therapy Association
http://www.amtamassage.org/
English

The Web site provides news of the American Massage Therapy Association, which aims to promote professional credibility, continuing education, and information resources in the massage therapy profession.

American Organization for Bodywork Therapies of Asia
http://www.aobta.org/
English

> The Web site provides news of the American Organization for Bodywork Therapies of Asia (AOBTA), which is a professional membership organization that promotes Asian Bodywork Therapy (ABT). AOBTA supports appropriate credentialing, definition of scopes of practice, and educational standards. AOBTA also promotes public education on the benefits, ethics, and principles of ABT.

American Tai Chi Association
http://www.americantaichi.org/pro.asp
English

> American Tai Chi Association aims to promote Tai Chi as a complementary and alternative medicine to benefit the public health and as a physical activity for fitness and wellness.

Qigong Institute
http://www.qigonginstitute.org/main_page/main_page.php
English

> The goals of the Qigong Institute are to promote medical Qigong via education, research, and clinical studies and to improve health care by integrating Qigong and Western medicine. It also has information on Qigong, especially as developed in China. Its Web site provides "What's New" and "Directory of Qigong Teachers/Therapists." It lists abstracts of Qigong PhD dissertations, scientific articles, reviews and other abstracts, which are available for public download. It also has a collection of "Qigong and Energy Medicine in the Press." There is a Qigong and Energy Medicine Database Online, which is a collection of over 3,500 abstracts collected by Dr. Sancier and the Qigong Institute over the past twenty years. However, users

have to pay in order to view the database online or to purchase the complete database on CD.

Qigong Research Society
http://www.qigongresearchsociety.com/
English

The Web site introduces Qigong therapy and Qigong exercise. It also provides news and course information.

Qi Gong Association of America
http://www.qi.org/
English

The Web site provides news and other Qigong articles and Qigong forums.

Tai Chi Union
http://www.taichiunion.com/
English

The Tai Chi Union for Great Britain aims to unite Taiji practitioners, to promote Taiji in all its aspects including health, aesthetic meditation, and self defense, and to improve standards and collate and disseminate information on Tai Chi classes and events in Great Britain and elsewhere. Selected articles published in *Tai Chi Chuan Magazine,* the union's publication, can be read on the Web site for free. It also provides many related links and much news.

Taijiquan and Qigong Federation for Europe
http://www.tcfe.org/
English

The Taijiquan and Qigong Federation for Europe was founded in 1997 as an organization that could bring together practitioners of Taiji quan and Qigong on the continent of Europe and to advance the practice of these Chinese internal arts. The federation holds a meeting every two years, and membership is open to European organizations. The TCFE Web site provides local contact information for TCFE organizations in all European countries in addition to news and events of interest. TCFE seeks participation and suggestions from both teachers and practitioners of Taiji quan and Qigong throughout Europe. The Web site provides news about Taiji quan and Qigong.

The National Qigong Association
http://www.nqa.org/
English

The National Qigong Association is a nonprofit organization of Qigong enthusiasts that work together to promote Qigong in America. It also supports those who are researching the benefits of Qigong. The Web site introduces Qigong and information of conferences held by the association. The association publishes *The Journal of Qigong in America,* and it provides many Qigong articles on its Web site.

The International Qigong Foundation for Social Oncology
http://www.socialoncology.com/
English

The Web site introduces the International Qigong Foundation for Social Oncology, Inc., which is a nonprofit foundation supporting educational programs in medical Qigong, Taiji quan, and yoga. It also introduces its activities, Qigong and social oncology. The goal of the foundation is to promote health or what the ancients described as "methods to eliminate diseases and prolong life."

CAM OR RELATED ORGANIZATIONS

Due to the vast amount of Web sites of CAM organizations, except for those that are exceptionally important, only the titles, URL and languages of a selected number of Web sites will be listed in this section.

Alternative Medicine Directory
http://www.shareguide.com/shdir1.html
English

Alternative medicine Directory
http://www.oohoi.com/health_dir/directory.htm
English

Alternative Medicine Foundation
http://www.amfoundation.org/
English

Alternative Therapies for Alcohol and Drug Abuse
http://nccam.nih.gov/training/centers/descriptions.htm#neuro1
English

> Center (of McLean Hospital/Harvard Medical School and funded by NACCM) investigators will evaluate whether two traditional Chinese herbal remedies and an electrical acupuncture technique can be used to prevent addiction relapse and craving for alcohol and drugs of abuse. The four interactive projects will encompass the biochemical and biological standardization and characterization of the herbal remedies, test their effect in vitro and in animals, and perform a clinical evaluation of efficacy. In addition, the effectiveness of the electroacupuncture technique in animals and human participants will be evaluated (Web site, NCCAM).

Association of Accredited Naturopathic Medical Colleges
http://www.aanmc.org/index.php
English

Bandolier
http://www.jr2.ox.ac.uk/Bandolier/
English

> Articles are provided for free. The Web site is intended to gather the best evidence available about complementary and alternative therapies for sufferers and professionals. It will be updated as more or better evidence becomes available and will be accessible over the Internet. It contains stories from Bandolier, plus abstracts of systematic reviews, meta-analyses, or other studies about CAT. By entering keywords like "acupuncture" and "Chinese medicine" in the search engine, users can search for related articles published on *Bandolier.*

Centre for Integrative Medicine
www.compmed.umm.edu/
English

Complementary and Alternative Healing University
http://alternativehealing.org/
English

Complementary Medical Association
http://www.the-cma.org.uk/default.aspx?id = 2909
English

General Complementary Medicine Organizations
 & Professional Bodies
http://www.bcma.co.uk/index.htm
English

**Geneva Foundation for Medical Education and Research-
Traditional medicine and Complementary/Alternative
medicine
http://www.gfmer.ch/TMCAM/TMCAM.htm
English, French, German, Spanish**

This is the Web site of the Centre for Research in Medical Bio-
climatology, Biotechnologies, and Natural Medicines of Milan
University, and the Geneva Foundation for Medical Education
and Research, WHO Collaborating Centre in Education and
Research in Human Reproduction. The Web site is divided into
three sections: "Medical Education," "Publication," and "Links."
"Medical Education" links to the teaching and training activities provided by Centre for Research in Medical Bioclimatol-
ogy, Biotechnologies, and Natural Medicines of Milan University. "Publication" links to list of articles written by experts in
English, Italian, or French. One of the titles "Traditional Medicine and Complementary/Alternative Medicine" by Dr. Hong-
guang Dong includes the following articles: "Acupuncture Consultation, Acupuncture for the Management of Dysmenorrhea,"
"Acupuncture in Gynecology and Obstetrics," " Acupuncture in
the Treatment of Amenorrhea," "Alternative Medicine and the
Perimenopause," "Conventional Medicine in Combination with
Acupuncture in the Treatment of Menopausal Symptoms," and
"Neurophysiology of Acupuncture." The Web site has links to
free medical journals, an atlas, books, dictionaries, guidelines
and organizations.

**Health on the Net Foundation
http://www.hon.ch/
English, French, and Spanish**

**Institute for Complementary Medicine
http://www.i-c-m.org.uk/
English**

Oregon Center for Complementary and Alternative Medicine in Neurological Disorders
http://www.ohsu.edu/orccamind/
English

Oriental Medicine Internet Resources
http://www.holisticmed.com/www/ormed.html
English

> The site offers a list of Oriental Medicine links. The links are divided into "Extensive Information & Meta-Directories," "National/International Organizations," "Practitioner Databases," "Web-Based Discussion Forums," "General Interest Pages," "Education & Training," "Publications," and "Oriental Medicine Discussion Groups."

Paradigm Media Center
http://www.paradigm-pubs.com/html/mediacenter.html
English

> The Web site introduces the Media Centre, which is a service to inform the public about acupuncture and Chinese medicine by providing information to make intelligent and informed choices about the available clinical options. The Web site is designed to provide easy access to references for basic information and to ad hoc materials that could be required by book reviewers and editors. The Web site includes "new releases," "references," "background papers on acupuncture and Chinese medicine," and "materials for book reviewers and bibliographers." "Background papers on acupuncture and Chinese medicine" provides the following titles: "Acupuncture Research with Questions and Answers," "Chinese Herbal Medicine," "Chinese Medicine Today," "The Ancient History of Chinese medicine," "The Modern History of Chinese Medicine."

Prince of Wales's Foundation for Integrated Health
http://www.fih.org.uk
English

Quackwatch
http://www.quackwatch.org/index.html
English

> Founded by Dr. Stephen Barrett in 1969, the Lehigh Valley Committee Against Health Fraud is a nonprofit corporation whose purpose is to combat health-related frauds, myths, fads, and fallacies. The organization assumed its current name, Quackwatch, Inc. in 1997. Its primary focus is on quackery-related information. The organization began developing a worldwide network of volunteers and expert advisors. Its activities include: investigating questionable claims; answering inquiries about products and services; advising quackery victims; distributing reliable publications; reporting illegal marketing; assisting or generating consumer-protection lawsuits; improving the quality of health information on the Internet; attacking misleading advertising on the Internet. The Web site challenges the validity of acupuncture, Chinese medicine, and Qigong therapy. It lists "Non-recommended Sources of Health Advice," which includes periodicals and Web sites relevant to Chinese medicine.

Research Council for Complementary Medicine
http://www.rccm.org.uk/
English

Start Group Index
http://www.itmonline.org/arts/startindex.htm#
English

Society of Integrative Medicine
http://www.mmsionline.com/intmed/
English

The Commission for Scientific Medicine and Mental Health
http://www.csmmh.org/
English

The Foundation for Chiropractic Education and Research
http://www.fcer.org/about.htm
English

WHO Collaborating Centres for Traditional Medicine
http://www.who.int/medicines/areas/traditional/collabcentres/
** en/index.html**
English, while Arabic, Chinese (Simplified), French, Russian,
** Spanish versions are currently unavailable**

> The Web site publishes WHO research reports on traditional medicine, including "WHO Traditional Medicine Strategy 2002-2005," "Definitions of Traditional Medicines Terms," and "WHO Collaborating Centres for Traditional Medicine." In the section of "Publication," there are research reports and use guideline for acupuncture and herbal medicines.

Chapter 3

Libraries

As the Internet expands its functions, the power of libraries' online catalogs grows stronger. In this chapter, two categories of libraries are introduced: universities or research institute libraries, and virtual libraries. The Web sites of universities or research institutes provide free online catalog searches. Usually there is an introduction to the traditional medicine database on the library's homepage. Moreover, some library Web sites offer additional services. For example, the library of Guangzhou University of TCM provides free "Video on Demand," in which seminars are recorded and put online for public view. Among the video clips available, many are lectures on Traditional Chinese Medicine. The library of Shanghai University of TCM also serves as an information center.

The East Asian Library of the University of Pittsburgh provides a very practical service. In cooperation with university libraries in Hong Kong and Taiwan, the library made photocopies of essays available for researchers in the United States free of charge. Other than university libraries, another category to be discussed in this chapter is virtual libraries, which charge fees. Although these Web sites are for commercial purposes, they are exceptionally convenient to use. Many of these virtual libraries have scanned a rich collection of Chinese manuscripts, and users can purchase these files and download them directly. These virtual libraries often have a massive collection on their user-friendly Web sites. Most of the libraries have thousands of titles on Traditional Chinese Medicine.

The following two Web sites are the two most popular virtual libraries in Mainland China. Books on Traditional Chinese Medicine could be found in the section titled "Medicine—Hygiene." Some of the books can be downloaded for free. The author attempted downloading a few titles from the Apabi and Superstar Digital libraries. The scanned pages are clear, and the Web sites are easy to use.

Apabi
http://apabi.nstl.gov.cn/dlib/List.asp
Chinese (simplified)

> Established by the National Science and Technology Library, Apabi is a virtual library that offers electronic books for a fee. Apabi contains over 1,000 titles written in Chinese on Traditional Chinese Medicine. A rich and varied collection. Only available in simplified Chinese. Users must have Apabi Reader, which can be downloaded from the page for free. "Chinese Medicine" is listed under the category *yiyao—weisheng* (Medicine—Hygiene), yet there is no further division, making the search more difficult.

Superstar Digital Library
http://www.ssreader.com/
Chinese (simplified)

> Superstar Digital Library is a virtual library based in Mainland China. It claims to be the largest Chinese virtual library in the world, which includes over 20,000 Chinese books. It also includes over 1,000 books on Chinese medicine published in Chinese. The section "Chinese medicine" is categorized into seventeen subjects.

Note: User friendly. A rich and varied collection. Only available in simplified Chinese. Users must have SSReader, which can be downloaded from the page for free.

UNIVERSITIES

The followings are the Web sites of TCM university libraries. Since most of these Web sites are similar, only the names of those libraries of the most respectable size are listed.

Beijing University of TCM Library
http://202.204.33.222/tpi_36/sysasp/include/index.asp
Chinese (simplified)

Chengdu University of Traditional Chinese Medicine Library
http://lib.cdutcm.edu.cn/
Chinese (simplified)

China Medical University Library, Taiwan
http://lib.cmu.edu.tw/~lib/
Chinese (traditional)

China Pharmaceutical University Library
http://lib.cpu.edu.cn
Chinese (simplified)

Guangzhou University of Traditional Chinese medicine Library
http://library.gzhtcm.edu.cn
Chinese (simplified)

The site also offers online videos about lectures held in the university.

Nanjing University of Traditional Chinese Medicine Library
http://lib.njutcm.edu.cn
Chinese (simplified)

Shandong University of Traditional Medicine Library
http://210.44.165.61/
Chinese (simplified)

Shanghai University of TCM Library
http://lib.shutcm.com
Chinese (simplified)

The majority of titles available in the university libraries are in Chinese. For materials in English, users may visit the library Web sites of the Middlesex University and the University of Westminster. Both universities provide regular TCM degree programs, and their libraries have a complete collection of traditional Chinese medical materials in English.

Middlesex University Library
http://www.lr.mdx.ac.uk/
English

University of Westminster Library
http://www.wmin.ac.uk/page-611
English

ORGANIZATIONS

The followings are Web sites of libraries from national organizations.

British Library
http://www.bl.uk/services/reading.html
English

The library provides photocopies of papers at approximately £5 per paper and access to medical databases including AMED, for life sciences, technologies, and humanities. It also manages interlibrary loans of theses and reports. Frequent users and those who are interested in borrowing material on a library-to-library basis can register for the service.

Library of China Academy of TCM
http://www.cintcm.ac.cn/xxs/jj-e.html
English

The site has a brief introduction of the library without any online service available.

Library of Chinese Academy Sciences
http://www.las.ac.cn/index.jsp
Chinese (simplified) and English

The library Web site offers an online catalog search and Internet guide for Chinese medicine, and it also introduces how to use online databases of Chinese medicine.

National Electronic Library for Health
http://www.library.nhs.uk/Default.aspx
English

In collaboration with NHS Libraries, the national electronic Library for Health Program is working to develop a digital library for NHS staff, patients, and the public. Through the search engine on the page, users can find information on Chinese medicine. The Headlines section also provides the latest research information on complementary and alternative medicine, including Chinese medicine.

National Library of China Online Electronic Library
http://www.nlc.gov.cn/GB/channel1/index.html
Chinese (simplified)

National Library of Medicine
http://www.nlm.nih.gov/
English

> The world's largest medical library, the National Library of Medicine (NLM), is located in the campus of the National Institutes of Health in Bethesda, Maryland. The library collects materials in all areas of biomedicine and health care and provides information and research services. It is the most important medical library Web site in the United States. It offers health information, a library catalog, online exhibition and digital project, and biomedical research resources. NLM also sets up many useful databases such as PubMed and MedlinePlus. NLM created "Current Bibliographies on Medicine-Acupuncture," which is a very useful guide to navigate on acupuncture.

National Science and Technology Library
http://www.nstl.gov.cn/index.html
Chinese (simplified)

> Established in 2000, National Science and Technology Library is a virtual information center that provides Chinese and English full-text articles and a dissertation delivery service for a fee. The site contains a journals and dissertations retrieval system that works in both Chinese and English.

Online Catalogue Center, National Library of China
http://olcc.nlc.gov.cn/
Chinese (simplified)

> A large online catalog for Chinese books.

PerioPath: Index to Chinese Periodical Literature (Chinese and English)
http://readopac2.ncl.edu.tw/ncl3/index.jsp
Chinese (traditional)

> PerioPath is an online index created and maintained by the National Central Library of Taiwan. It contains information on approximately 2,600 articles written in Chinese and Western language published on periodicals in Taiwan, Hong Kong, and Macau from 1994. Users can search for articles under title, author, class code, keyword, journal title, or publication date. The database contains twenty-five Chinese medical journals published in Taiwan.

Other useful library Web sites:

Cathay Herbal Library
http://www.cathayherbal.com/library/index.htm
English

> The Web site, established by Cathay Herbal Laboratories Pty Ltd., is a company that sells patented Chinese medicine. It offers comprehensive information on Traditional Chinese Herbal Medicine on the Web for both Western doctors and Traditional Chinese Medicine practitioners.

Copac Academic & National Library Catalogue
http://www.copac.ac.uk
English

> The Copac Academic & National Library Catalogue is a union catalog that provides a merged catalog of twenty-four major university research libraries in the United Kingdom and Ireland, including the British Library. It also includes the catalogs of special collections such as the National Art Library.

East Asian History of Science Library
http://www.nri.org.uk/library.html
English

The East Asian History of Science Library is the library of the Needham Research Institute. The first collections in the library were assembled both in China and the Western world from 1937 onward by Joseph Needham and Lu Gwei-Djen for the Science and Civilization in China (SCC) project. The library continues to expand its collection to further the research on Science and Civilization of East Asia. The library houses a large collection of primary and secondary works on the history of traditional East Asian science, technology, and medicine written in Chinese, English, Korean, Japanese, and other languages. The library holds offprint, serials, and unpublished manuscripts regarding Traditional Chinese Medicine and the history of Chinese medicine. The site offers instructions to search the Online Public Access Catalogue of Cambridge University library. Moreover, the library also holds lectures, text-reading seminars, and conferences frequently.

Finding Information for Chinese Medicine, RMIT
http://www.lib.rmit.edu.au/guides/chinese-medicine.html
English

This Web site lists TCM books and online resources of the RMIT Library. It serves as a guide to supply tips for finding information on Chinese medicine. It also lists relevant resources accessible at RMIT University Library.

Gateway Service Center of Chinese Academic Journal
 Publications
http://www.library.pitt.edu/gateway/
English

The Gateway Service Center is administered by the East Asian Library of the University of Pittsburgh Library System. Its objectives are to provide free delivery of full-text Chinese-language academic publications to any researcher who cannot find the needed item in U.S. libraries. Indeed, any user who needs articles related to Chinese medicine published in Chinese may use the service. Participating libraries in Mainland China, Hong Kong, and Taiwan, where the titles are held, will transmit full-text articles electronically via the Internet.

The Web site provides very helpful service.

How to Find Information on TCM
http://link.library.utoronto.ca/eal/flash/resource_guides.cfm
  ?id = 23
English

This Web site, created by Cheng Yu Tung East Asian Library of University of Toronto, provides a brief introduction to some principal sources in Chinese medicine based on the library's collection.

Library Databases for Herbs, Spices & Medicinal Plants
http://www.library.umass.edu/instruction/tutorials/herbs/
  databases.html
English

The Web site, created by the library of the University of Massachusetts, offers annotations on databases related to herbs and medicinal plants. It is a very good starting point to know more about herbs.

Image Collection of Old Medical Book, Kyushu University
  Library
http://herakles.lib.kyushu-u.ac.jp/icomb/index-e.html
Japanese and English

Held by the Medical Library of Kyushu University, it is one of the greatest Japanese collections of Eastern and Western medical books and manuscripts. Since the spring of 2003, images of books and manuscripts from this database have been put together into a pictorial database, in order to facilitate study and general interest in the history of medicine. Currently, the database holds more than 9,000 images from about 300 manuscripts and books, and each image is available in both standard quality version and high-quality version (over 300dpi), for computer display and printing, respectively. Users can search on the English Web site with keywords like "acupuncture" and "massage." Every book is listed with detailed information of its publication. The quality of the scanned images is high.

Institute of Medical Information/Medical Library
http://www.library.imicams.ac.cn/index.aspx
Chinese (simplified)

The library has plenty of resources (such as catalogs and databases) about medical sciences, including Chinese medicine.

Kyoto University Library Fujikawa Database
http://edb.kulib.kyoto-u.ac.jp/exhibit/fuji/index.html
Japanese

Fujikawa is a famous Japanese medical historian. Kyoto University houses Fujikawa's book collection, comprised of medical literature. The books are scanned and listed on the Web site with introductions to every title.

NoWAL (North West Academic Libraries)
http://www.nowal.ac.uk
English

An association of all libraries in universities and colleges in Cheshire, Cumbria, Greater Manchester, Lancashire, and Merseyside in the United Kingdom, NoWAL aims to enhance the delivery of library services to the higher education community in northwest United Kingdom. It provides services like design and delivery of staff training courses, a reciprocal access and borrowing policy, and a consortia procurement of library materials.

NCPC New Drug Research and Development Co., Ltd Library
http://www.ncpcrd.com.cn/lib/
Chinese (simplified)

Established by NCPC New Drug Research and Development Co. Ltd, the library Web site provides the following journals: *Chinese Traditional Patent Medicine, Journal of Beijing University of Traditional Chinese Medicine, Chinese Journal of Integration Traditional and Western Medicine,* and *Northwest Pharmaceutical Journal.* The site also introduces other useful Web sites related to Chinese medicine.

Pharmaceutical Digital Library
http://www.pharmadl.com/pharmadl/index.aspx
English

Established by the Institute of Medical Industry Information Center, the library Web site aims to offer medical information, databases, and consultation services. After registration, readers may read Chinese pharmaceutical news, search the databases, and read the full-text journals published by the institute, such as *Zhongguo yiyao gongye za zhi* (Chinese journal of pharmaceuticals).

Sinological Serials in European Libraries Project
http://sun.sino.uni-heidelberg.de/sselp/index.html
English

Established by the European Association of Chinese Studies, Sinological Serials in European Libraries Project (SSELP) is a database of sinological and Chinese-language serials in European collections. Its objective is to locate periodicals and serials of Chinese studies throughout Europe and to provide a tool for improving research and communication between institutes and other learned societies. Chinese-language periodicals of other fields are also recorded. It searches Chinese medical materials in European libraries only.

European Virtual OPAC for Chinese Studies
http://www.sino.uni-heidelberg.de/evocs/
English

The database is an easy way to search the holdings of major sinological libraries in Europe. One can search it by Western languages, Romanized Japanese, and Korean and Romanized Chinese.

TCM Herb Library
http://www.rmhiherbal.org/ai/pharintro.html
English

Established by Rocky Mountain Herbal Institute, TCM Herb Library provides free access (by password) to sample course materials and a database of over 290 herbs of the Chinese (TCM) *Materia Medica*. After registration, users may access the herb library, textbook of traditional Chinese herbal sciences, and herbal database for free.

TCM Resources at HKUST Library
http://library.ust.hk/guides/tcm/tcm-ust.html
Chinese (traditional) and English

The site lists all electronic and printed information sources on Traditional Chinese Medicine at HKUST Library. Although HKUST does not have Chinese medicine courses, it develops the research of Chinese medicine. This subject guide focuses on *Materia Medica* and pharmacognosy. It has also selected some of the best TCM sites on the Internet. Web site contents include bibliographies, comprehensive treatises, databases, dictionaries, encyclopedia, formulae and prescriptions, handbooks and manuals, illustrations and identification, periodicals, and reports.

The Internet Health Library
http://www.Internethealthlibrary.com/
English

A free independent service, the Internet Health Library, provides its users with access to news, research, and information relating to health and well-being. It also introduces alternative and complementary therapies and natural health care resources. The service aims to provide its users with the information required to make an informed choice about health and how to help themselves safely, naturally, and effectively with natural remedies. The Web site is updated daily with the latest information on diet, nutrition, and lifestyle. It also lists associations and organizations of Complementary and Alternative Medicine in the United Kingdom. Users may register for its free newsletter. The site is in association with the Department of Complementary Medicine, University of Exeter.

Traditional Chinese Medicine
http://w2.vu.edu.au/library/infolink/health/tcm2.htm
English

The Web site is established by Victoria University Library. It provides TCM resources and links. It contains all TCM books and journals collected in the Victoria University Library, together with other sections like "web reference tools," "electronic guides and handbooks," "general sites," "Chinese herbal medicine," "complementary therapies," "web organizations" and "web documents." The information collected is very comprehensive.

Wellcome Library
http://library.wellcome.ac.uk/
English

Wellcome Trust is an independent charity organization that supports research on biomedical science and history of medicine. Its library houses one of the world's greatest collections of books, manuscripts, archives, films, and paintings on the history of medicine from the earliest times to the present day. The site provides online catalogs, electronic resources, collections, exhibitions and projects. The catalog contains records for all Wellcome Library collections and material types. It covers both the history of medicine and current biomedical science topics. As well as books and journals, it is possible to retrieve entries for pictures, films, video and archives.

Chapter 4

Schools

TCM schools are the bases for Chinese medical education and research. Many TCM schools in Mainland China have Web sites with rich contents. Other than introducing programs and teachers' qualifications, these Web sites often present TCM-related news, conference announcements, research achievements, published works, etc., and most Web sites have English versions available. For example, the Web site of Guangxi Traditional Chinese Medical University provides much TCM-related news.

In 2003 the Ministry of Education of the People's Republic of China launched an initiative entitled *Jing pin ke cheng* (JPKC) (China's Higher Education Classic Course or China's Quality Opencourse-Ware).[1] To promote high-quality university-level online education, the Ministry of Education makes a certain number of courses available through *Jing pin ke cheng* every year. Free, searchable access to course materials is made available to educators, students, and those pursuing independent study around the world. (It should be noted that all JPKC courses are taught in Chinese with Mandarin as the spoken teaching medium.)

Of the three sets of courses that have been launched to date, three started in 2003, four in 2004, and five in 2005. Since the selection process is extremely rigorous and the number of courses taught in China terrifically large, it is a great honor for courses to be chosen as a JPKC. In fact, many universities invest considerable effort in preparing their submissions. In addition, some provinces and cities, such as Heilongjiang, Hunan, Beijing, and Shanghai, have launched their own JPKC initiatives.[2] In order to have their courses listed, universities have carefully designed their courses, utilizing multimedia teaching tools, and opening up their Web sites for public access. For example, Shanghai University of Traditional Chinese Medicine has put six of the courses submitted to JPKC online. It is anticipated that more and more courses will be available online.

All of the Chinese medicine courses presented via JPKC are taught by a group of teachers. The review process guarantees that content is reliable and comprehensive. Without a doubt, these Web sites provide the best way to study Chinese medicine for free. A list of the available courses follows: Diagnostics of Traditional Chinese Medicine[3] and Chinese Traditional Medicine[4] of Beijing University of Traditional Chinese Medicine; Herbal Prescription,[5] Chemistry of Traditional Chinese Medicine;[6] Synopsis of Prescriptions of the Golden Chamber[7] and Authentication of Chinese Medicines[8] of Heilongjiang University of Chinese Medicine; Wen-Bing[9] and Pediatrics of Traditional Chinese Medicine[10] of Nanjing University of Traditional Chinese Medicine; Acupuncture[11] and Experimental Traditional Chinese Medicine[12] of Shanghai University of Traditional Chinese Medicine; Traditional Chinese Gynecology[13] of Guangzhou University of Traditional Chinese Medicine; and Basic Theory of Traditional Chinese Medicine[14] of Liaoning University for Traditional Chinese Medicine.

The following is a list of TCM schools' Web sites collected by the author. Users should pay special attention to schools in Europe and North America.[15] If you are looking for a TCM program or a TCM practitioner, please choose carefully because the quality of these TCM schools varies. Users are suggested to seek for professional advice when choosing a TCM school.

GREATER CHINA (CHINA, TAIWAN, HONG KONG, AND MACAU)

Anhui College of Traditional Chinese Medicine
(Anhui zhong yi xue yuan 安徽中醫學院**)**
http://www.ahtcm.edu.cn/

Beijing University of Chinese Medicine
(Beijing zhong yi yao da xue 北京中醫藥大學**)**
http://www.bjucmp.edu.cn/

Graduate Institute of Traditional Chinese Medicine, College
of Medicine, Chang Gung University
(Changgeng da xue chuan tong Zhongguo yi xue yan jiu yuan
長庚大學傳統中國醫學研究院**)**
http://www.cgu.edu.tw/

Changchun University of Traditional Chinese Medicine
(Changchun zhong yi xue yuan 長春中醫學院**)**
http://www.ccutcm.com.cn/

Chengdu University of T.C.M.
(Chengdu zhong yi yao da xue 成都中醫藥大學**)**
http://www.cdutcm.edu.cn/

Emei College of Chengdu University of T. C. M.
(Chengdu zhong yi yao da xue Emei xue yuan 成都中醫藥大學
峨眉學院**)**
http://www.emtcm.com/

Fujian University of Traditional Chinese Medicine
(Fujian zhong yi yao xue yuan 福建中醫學院**)**
http://www.fjtcm.edu.cn/

Gansu College of Traditional Chinese Medicine
(Gansu zhong yi xue yuan 甘肅中醫學院**)**
http://www.gszy.edu.cn/

Guangxi Traditional Chinese Medical University
(Guangxi zhong yi xue yuan 廣西中醫學院)
http://www.gxtcmu.edu.cn/

Guangzhou University of Chinese Medicine (Previously
Guangzhou University of TCM)
(Guangzhou zhong yi yao da xue 廣州中醫藥大學)
http://www.gzhtcm.edu.cn/

GuiYang College of Traditional Chinese Medicine
(Guiyang zhong yi xue yuan 貴陽中醫學院)
http://www.gytcm.com/

Heilongjiang University of Chinese Medicine
(Heilongjiang zhong yi yao da xue 黑龍江中醫藥大學)
http://www.hljucm.net/

Henan College of TCM
(Henan zhong yi xue yuan 河南中醫學院)
http://www.hactcm.edu.cn/

Hubei College of Traditional Chinese Medicine
(Hubei zhong yi xue yuan 湖北中醫學院)
http://www.hbtcm.edu.cn/

Hunan University of Traditional Chinese Medicine
(Hunan zhong yi yao da xue 湖南中醫藥大學)
http://www.hnctcm.com/

Jiangxi University of Traditional Chinese Medicine
(Jiangxi zhong yi xue yuan 江西中醫學院)
http://www.jxtcmi.com/

Liaoning University of Traditional Chinese Medicine
(Liaoning zhong yi xue yuan 遼寧中醫學院)
http://www.lnutcm.edu.cn/

Nanjing University of Traditional Chinese Medicine
(Nanjing zhong yi yao da xue 南京中醫藥大學)
http://www.njutcm.edu.cn

Shaanxi University of Chinese Medicine
(Shaanxi zhong yi xue yuan 陝西中醫學院)
http://www.sntcm.edu.cn/

Shandong University of Traditional Chinese Medicine
(Shandong zhong yi yao da xue 山東中醫藥大學)
http://www.sdutcm.edu.cn/

Shanghai University of T.C.M.
(Shanghai zhong yi yao da xue 上海中醫藥大學)
http://www.shutcm.edu.cn/

Shanxi University of Traditional Chinese Medicine
(Shanxi zhong yi xue yuan 山西中醫藥大學)
http://www.sxtcm.com/

Sichuan Academy of Traditional Chinese Medicine
(Sichuan sheng zhong yi yao yan jiu yuan 四川省中醫藥研究院)
http://www.sczyy.org.cn/hthl.htm

The WEB based Acupuncture and Moxibustion
(Shanghai zhong yi yao da xue zhen jiu tui na xue yuan 上海中
醫藥大學針灸推拿學院)
http://www.acumox.org/zj_demo/

Tianjin University of Traditional Chinese Medicine
(Tianjin zhong yi xue yuan 天津中醫學院)
http://www.tjutcm.edu.cn/

Yunnan University of Traditional Chinese Medicine
(Yunnan zhong yi xue yuan 雲南中醫學院)
http://www.ynutcm.edu.cn/

Zhejiang Chinese Medical University
(Zhejiang zhong yi yao da xue 浙江中醫藥大學**)**
http://www.zjtcm.net/

China Pharmaceutical University
(Zhongguo yi yao ke da xue 中國藥科大學**)**
http://www.cpu.edu.cn/

School of Chinese Medicine, Hong Kong Baptist University
(香港浸會大學中醫學院)
http://www.hkbu.edu.hk/~scm/index/chi/index.html

School of Chinese Medicine, Chinese University of Hong Kong
(香港中文大學中醫學院)
http://www.cuhk.edu.hk/scm/

School of Chinese Medicine, University of Hong Kong
(香港大學中醫學院)
http://www3.hku.hk/chinmed/2005/Chinese/index.php

Faculty of Chinese Medicine, Macau University of Science
and Technology
(澳門科技大學中醫學院)
http://www.must.edu.mo/

China Academy of Chinese Medical Sciences
(Zhongguo zhong yi ke xue yuan 中國中醫科學院**)**
http://www.catcm.ac.cn/

Institute of Acupuncture and Moxibustion China Academy
of Chinese Medical Sciences
(Zhongguo zhong yi zhen jiu yan jiu suo 中國中醫針灸研究所**)**
http://iam.acutimes.com/

China Medical University, College of Chinese Medicine Taiwan
(中國醫藥大學中醫學院)
http://www2.cmu.edu.tw/~cchimed/

NORTH AMERICA (UNITED STATES AND CANADA)

Academy for Five Element Acupuncture
http://www.acupuncturist.edu/

Academy of Chinese Culture and Health Sciences
http://www.acchs.edu/

Academy of Classical Oriental Sciences
http://www.acos.org/

Academy of Oriental Medicine at Austin
http://www.aoma.edu

Acupuncture and Integrative Medicine College, Berkeley
http://www.aimc.edu/

Acupuncture and Massage College
http://www.amcollege.edu/

Alberta College of Acupuncture and Traditional Chinese Medicine
http://www.acatcm.com/

American College of Acupuncture and Oriental Medicine
http://www.acaom.edu/

American College of Traditional Chinese Medicine
http://www.actcm.org/

Arizona School of Acupuncture & Oriental Medicine
http://www.asaom.edu/

Atlantic University of Chinese Medicine
http://www.aucm.com/

Bastyr University, School of Acupuncture and Oriental Medicine
http://www.studyacupuncture.com/

Canadian College of Acupuncture and Oriental Medicine
http://www.ccaom.com/

Canadian College of Holistic Health (CCHH Diploma Programs)
http://www.cchh.org/
http://www.cchh.org/content.asp?MenuID = 3&SubMenuID =
7&incid = list&DepartmentID = 1&
CourseType = Program&ItemID = 23

Central College
http://www.centralcollege.ca/index1_ch.html

Chinese Healing Arts Center
http://www.qihealer.com

College de Rosemont, Departement d'acupuncture
http://www.agora.crosemont.qc.ca/dacu/

Colorado School of Traditional Chinese Medicine
http://www.cstcm.edu/

Dongguk Royal University
http://dru.edu/dru/eng/index.php

Dragon Rises College of Oriental Medicine
http://www.dragonrises.net/

East West College of Natural Medicine
http://www.ewcollege.org/

The University of East West Medicine
http://www.uewm.edu/

Eastern School of Acupuncture and Traditional Medicine
http://www.easternschool.com/

Edgewood College of Georgia School of Oriental Medicine
http://www.edgewood-college.com/

Emperor's College of Traditional Oriental Medicine
http://www.emperors.edu/

Five Branches Institute
http://www.fivebranches.edu

Florida College of Integrative Medicine
http://www.fcim.edu

Grant MacEwan College
http://www1.macewan.ca/web/hcs/acupuncture/home/index
    .cfm

Institute of Acupuncture & Traditional Chinese Medicine
http://www.recorder.ca/acupuncture/

Institute of Clinical Acupuncture and Oriental Medicine
http://www.orientalmedicine.edu/

Institute of Chinese Herbology Programs in Chinese Herbology
http://www.ich-herbschool.com/

International Academy of Medical Acupuncture
http://www.iama.edu/

International College of Traditional Chinese Medicine
    of Vancouver
http://www.tcmcollege.com/index.html

International College of Traditional Chinese Medicine Victoria
http://www.tcminternational.com/

Jung Tao School of Classical Chinese Medicine
http://www.jungtao.com/

Kansas College of Chinese Medicine
http://www.kccm.edu/

Medboo
http://www.ontcm.com/

Mercy College: Program in Acupuncture and Oriental Medicine
http://www.mercy.edu/index.cfm

Midwest College of Oriental Medicine
http://www.acupuncture.edu/midwest/index.html

National College of Natural Medicine
http://www.ncnm.edu/

Natural Healers (Portal for Searching Practitioners)
http://www.naturalhealers.com/

New England School of Acupuncture
http://www.nesa.edu

New York College of Health Professions
http://www.nycollege.edu/

New York College of Traditional Chinese Medicine
http://www.nyctcm.edu/

Northwestern Health Sciences University, Minnesota College of Acupuncture and Oriental Medicine
http://www.nwhealth.edu/

Ontario College of Traditional Chinese Medicine
http://www.octcm.com/

Oregon School of Oriental Medicine
http://www.ocom.edu/index.php

Oshio College of Acupuncture & Herbology
http://members.shaw.ca/oshio/

Pacific College of Oriental Medicine
http://www.pacificcollege.edu/

PCU College of Holistic Medicine
http://www.vcc-tcm.ca/chinese/index.html#shine

Phoenix Institute of Herbal Medicine & Acupuncture
http://pihma.edu/

Samra University of Oriental Medicine
http://www.samra.edu/

Santa Barbara College of Oriental Medicine
http://www.sbcom.edu/

Seattle Institute of Oriental Medicine
http://www.siom.com/

Shang Hai TCM College of B.C.
http://www.acupuncture-college.com/home.shtml

South Baylo University
http://www.southbaylo.edu/

Southern California University of Health Sciences
http://www.scuhs.edu/

Southwest Acupuncture College
http://www.acupuncturecollege.edu/

Swedish Institute, College of Health Sciences
http://www.swedishinstitute.org/

Tai Sophia Institute for the Healing Arts
http://www.tai.edu/

Texas College of Traditional Chinese Medicine
http://www.texastcm.edu

The American Academy of Acupuncture and Oriental Medicine
http://www.aaaom.edu

The East-West School of Chinese Medicine
http://east-west.co.il/pageEnglish.asp

Toronto School of Traditional Chinese Medicine
http://www.tstcm.com/

Traditional Chinese Medical College of Hawaii
http://www.tcmch.edu/

Tri-state College of Acupuncture
http://www.tsca.edu/

University of Bridgeport, Acupuncture Institute
http://www.bridgeport.edu/pages/3247.asp

University of Maryland, Medical Center
http://www.umm.edu/

World Medicine Institute
http://www.acupuncture-hi.com/

Yo San University of TCM
http://www.yosan.edu/

EUROPE AND AUSTRALIA

Acupuncture Foundation
http://www.acupuncturefoundation.com/

Australian College of Natural Medicine
http://www.acnm.edu.au/

Australian Institute of Applied Sciences
http://www.aias.com.au/

College of Integrated Chinese Medicine
http://www.cicm.org.uk/

European University of Chinese Medicine
http://www.eucm.org/

London College of Traditional Acupuncture and Oriental Medicine
http://www.lcta.com

School of Health and Social Sciences, Middlesex University
http://www.mdx.ac.uk/

Northern College of Acupuncture
http://www.chinese-medicine.co.uk/

New Zealand School of Acupuncture and Traditional Chinese Medicine
http://www.acupuncture.co.nz/

Renshu College of Chinese Medicine
http://www.renshu.ac.uk/

Division of Chinese Medicine, RMIT University
http://www.rmit.edu.au/chinese-med

The College of Chinese Medicine
http://www.thecollegeofchinesemedicine.com/

The College of Traditional Chinese Medicine, University of Technology Sydney
http://www.science.uts.edu.au/centres/tcm/courses.html

School of Biomedical Sciences, University of Western Sydney
http://www.uws.edu.au/about/acadorg/schools/
biomedicalsciences

School of Integrated Health, University of Westminster
http://www.wmin.ac.uk/sih/

Sydney Institute of Traditional Chinese Medicine
http://www.sitcm.edu.au/

School of Health Sciences, Victoria University
http://www.vu.edu.au/

The Scottish School of Herbal Medicine
http://www.herbalmedicine.org.uk/rootpages/teaching.shtml

Southern School of Natural Therapies
http://www.southernschool.com/

International College of Oriental Medicine
http://www.orientalmed.ac.uk/

The Acupuncture Foundation, Ireland
http://www.acupuncturefoundation.org/

NOTES

1. Jing Pin Ke Cheng URL: http://166.111.180.5/new. An article introduces the detailed courses on Chinese medicine included in JPKC. Ka wai

FAN, "Chinese Medicine Courses on the Internet," *The Journal of Alternative and Complementary Medicine, 13*,7, 2007 pp. 777-780.

2. http://166.111.180.5/new/test/test.asp.
3. http://jpkc.bjucmp.edu.cn/zhongyizhenduan/05.1.13/1.htm.
4. http://jpkc.bjucmp.edu.cn/zhongyaoxue/main.htm.
5. http://www.hljucm.net/web_cai/guojia/fjx/index.htm.
6. http://www.hljucm.net/web_cai/guojia/zyhx/index.htm.
7. http://www.hljucm.net/web_cai/0507jgyl.htm.
8. http://www.hljucm.net/web_cai/zyjd/index.htm.
9. http://202.195.210.110/wb/.
10. http://202.195.210.110/erk/.
11. http://www.acumox.org/zj_demo/.
12. http://jpkc.shutcm.edu.cn/syzyx/.
13. http://210.38.96.15:8080/guojia/index.htm.
14. http://jp.lnutcm.edu.cn/zhongji/.

15. The latest introduction to Chinese medicine in Western countries, please see "Chinese Medicine Education in Australia," "Chinese Medicine Education in New Zealand," "Chinese Medicine Education in Norway," "Chinese Medicine Education in the UK" "Chinese Medicine Education in the USA" "Chinese Medicine Education in Canada." In Michael McCarthy (ed.) (2007). *Thieme Almanac: Acupuncture and Chinese Medicine. Thieme Almanac: Acupuncture and Chinese Medicine,* tuttgart: Thieme, pp. 208-228.

Chapter 5

Journals

Chinese medicine has gained increasing recognition around the world for its role in the prevention and treatment of diseases, and spending on professional Chinese medical services has increased substantially. Chinese medicine continues to gain ground on conventional medicine, which is dominated by Western science. In addition, serious research on Chinese medicine, whether written in English or Chinese, has been published in peer-reviewed journals. Therefore, it is both important and useful for scholars and amateurs to familiarize themselves with the Web sites of journals on Chinese medicine. Science Citation Index also includes the category of Integrative and Complementary Medicine for CAM journals and their impact factors can be found.

GENERAL

Abstract and Review of Clinical Traditional Chinese Medicine
http://www.rmhiherbal.org/hscc/#absrev
English

Published between 1991 and 1996—now ceased publication. The Web site lists only the tables of contents of past issues. Past issues can be purchased on the Web site.

American Journal of Chinese Medicine
http://www.worldscinet.com/ajcm/ajcm.shtml
English

Jointly published by the World Scientific Publishing Company and Tang Center for Herbal Medicine Research, University of Chicago, this journal publishes articles related to TCM and ethnomedicine. Articles include topics such as: basic scientific and clinical research in indigenous medical techniques, therapeutic procedures, medicinal plants, and traditional medical theories and concepts; multidisciplinary studies of medical practice and health care; international policy implications of comparative studies of medicine in all cultures; and translating scholarly ancient texts or modern publications on ethnomedicine.

American Journal of Traditional Chinese Medicine
http://www.bloominglotus.net/journal.html
English

Published and managed by Blooming Lotus, Inc., this is the official journal of the Traditional Chinese Medicine Association and Alumni. According to the journal's Web site, the aims of the journal are: to provide accurate and up-to-date information on TCM, both academic and theoretical; and to promote the development of TCM in the United States; to promote better communication between TCM practitioners and allied health care practitioners, and to provide TCM practitioners with more scientifically based information with which to guide their practice. The tables of contents of volumes 1 to 7 are available online.

Asian Medicine: Tradition and Modernity
http://www.brill.nl/m_catalogue_sub6_id22461.htm
English

Aimed at researchers and practitioners of Asian Medicine in Asia as well as in Western countries, this is a multidisciplinary journal on Asian medicine and practice reports from clinicians.

It publishes academic articles from various areas, such as history, anthropology, archaeology, sociology, and philology. It will be of relevance to those studying the modifications and adaptations of traditional medical systems on their progression to non-Asian settings and will also be relevant to those who wish to learn more about the traditional background and practice of Asian medicine within its countries of origin. *Asian Medicine* has been published annually since 2005.

Australian Journal of Acupuncture and Chinese Medicine
http://www.acupuncture.org.au/ajacm.cfm
English

As the official Journal of the Australian Acupuncture and Chinese Medicine Association Ltd., this is Australia's peer-reviewed journal for the acupuncture and Chinese medicine profession. It publishes articles and essays related to acupuncture and Chinese medicine clinical practice and/or research and to stimulate the exchange of ideas about clinical practice and the role of acupuncture and Chinese medicine in contemporary health care. The journal has been published bi-annually since 2007. The Web site is still under construction. It has an author's guide, but provides no index or sample issue.

Beijing Traditional Chinese Medicine
http://210.77.146.154:8080/iTCMedu/bjzyzz/index.jsp
Chinese (Simplified)

The Web site offers the index and complete text of volume 12, published in 2004. Other contents can be read after registration. The Web site does not provide other information.

Blue Poppy Online Journal
http://www.bluepoppy.com/client_login/index.cfm
English

This site publishes articles for non-Chinese readers. The site offers many free articles for public download. Once registered, users receive free essays through e-mail. Each quarterly issue includes approximately thirty articles on a wide range of subjects from modern Chinese research literature. The journal sorts through Chinese journals and provides extracts from those articles most relevant to practice in the West.

Blue Poppy also provides research reports and information about acupuncture needles, books, and herbal products.

California Journal of Oriental Medicine
http://www.csomaonline.org/i4a/pages/index.cfm?pageid =
  3289
English

Published by the California State Oriental Medicine Association, this site publishes articles covering research, clinical therapies, and historical data in Oriental medicine. It is a bi-annual journal. Contents and abstracts from the journal are not available online.

Chinese Journal of Information on Traditional Chinese
  Medicine
http://www.cintcm.ac.cn/xxs/journal-e.html
English

Sponsored by the State Administration of Traditional Chinese Medicine and published by the National TCM Information and Library Coordination Committee and the Institute of Information on TCM of the China Academy of Traditional Chinese Medicine, this journal offers analyses and reports on new policies, trends, progresses, achievements, inventions, technologies, therapies, as well as new thoughts and market opportunities in the field of Traditional Chinese Medicine. It contains topics such as clinical work, research, administration and management, production, sales and marketing, and teaching. It includes columns on special topic forums, policies and laws, regulations, reform and management, research and prospects, scientific research trends, academic trends, educational trends, TCM research and development, selected clinical reports, current refractory diseases, nondrug therapies, achievements and patents, ethnic medicine, medical stars, domestic markets, TCM abroad, international markets, windows on Taiwan, Hong Kong, and Macao, the network world, and classified TCM information in China.

Chinese Journal of Integrated Traditional and Western Medicine
http://zxyjh.periodicals.net.cn/default.html
Chinese (simplified)

Managed by the China Association for Science and Technology, and organized by the Chinese Association of Integrative Medicine, it covers integrative medicine in China. It mainly concerns government policies on TCM and the integration of traditional and Western medicine. It publishes articles and reports, including clinical medicine, scientific research, preventive methods, and educational measures undertaken on integrated traditional and Western medicine. Its aims to enhance the integration of traditional and Western medicine and to advance the modernization of medicine in China.

Chinese Medical Journal
http://www.cmj.org/
Chinese (simplified) and English

Published by the *Chinese Medical Journal,* this is a peer-reviewed medical journal targeted at doctors, researchers, and health workers. Established in 1887, it is the oldest medical periodical in China and is distributed worldwide. Its highly informative Web site offers medical news, medical conferences, brief reports, case reports, and original articles. Current and past issues are also provided free of charge.

Chinese Medical Sciences Journal
http://www.tandf.co.uk/journals/titles/10019294.asp
English

Published by the Chinese Academy of Medical Sciences, this provides original research papers, review papers, and short communications on all aspects of basic and clinical medicine, pharmacology, and TCM. A free sample copy is available.

Chinese Medicine
http://www.cmjournal.org/
English

Published by Biomed Central, *Chinese Medicine* is the official journal of the International Society for Chinese Medicine, and all articles are open to the public. Its Web site publishes only the journal's first issue.

European Journal of Oriental Medicine
http://www.ejom.co.uk/
English

The *European Journal of Oriental Medicine* is the journal of the British Acupuncture Council. It aims to stimulate debate and scholarship in Chinese medicine and other traditions of Oriental medicine, creative interchange, and critical reflection. It publishes articles not only related to clinical practice but also wider topics including education, philosophy, politics, and medical anthropology. Each issue is themed to attract diverse contributions from both practitioners and academics. It publishes articles about Chinese medicine and other traditions of Oriental medicine. Abstracts of current and back issues are available.

Hunan Guiding Journal of Traditional Chinese Medicine and Pharmacology
http://210.77.146.154:8080/iTCMedu/hnzyzz/index.jsp
Chinese (simplified)

On the Web site are many essays that are published in the journal, with English abstracts. Users can search essays published between 2003 and 2007 through the search engine on the site.

The connection is rather unstable. Users are disconnected frequently.

Internet Journal of the Institute for Traditional Medicine
http://www.itmonline.org/journal
English

Published by the Institute for Traditional Medicine on the Internet, this can be accessed free of charge. Only six downloadable articles are available on the Web site. The Web site has not been updated since 2002. It is uncertain whether the journal has ceased publications.

Jiangsu Journal of Traditional Chinese Medicine
http://www.jstcm.cn/ch/index.aspx
Chinese (simplified)

This journal has many special columns such as "Special report," "Commissioned feature," "The avenue of the renowned physicians," "Doctors' Chat Room," "Academic investigation," "Experiences of experienced physicians," "Clinical report," "The physicians' roundtable," "Acupuncture and Tuina," "TCM education," "Experiments and research," etc. Its Web site provides the index of the current issue. Users can read the complete text only after registering.

Jiangxi Journal of Traditional Chinese Medicine
http://www.jxtcmi.com/xuebao/
Chinese (simplified)

The Web site only gives an introduction to each issue and provides the tables of contents of all issues published in 2003.

Journal for the Japan Society for Oriental Medicine
http://www.jsom.or.jp/html/magazine.htm
English and Japanese

Published by the Japan Society for Oriental Medicine, this Web site provides the index of issues published between 1999 and 2007.

Journal of Chinese Medicine
http://www.jcm.co.uk/
English

Publishes articles on all aspects of Chinese medicine, both theoretically and clinically, including acupuncture, Chinese herbal medicine, dietary medicine, medical Qigong, and Chinese medical history and philosophy. Sample articles are available on the Web site. In JCM's archive, articles are categorized under "acupuncture points," "acupuncture techniques," "case histories," "diseases," "general discussion," "general theory," "health preservation," "herbal medicine," and "history and massage." Complete articles can be purchased individually.

The Web site established *The Journal of Chinese Medicine Discussion Forum,* providing professionals with a platform for discussion.

Journal of Oriental Medicine and the Pain Clinic
http://www.osaka-med.ac.jp/~ane013/TOPEINDEX.html#B
English and Japanese

Published by the research society of Oriental Medicine and by the Pain Clinic of Japan. Indexes of each issue published from 1971 to 1998 are available online.

Journal of the Australian Traditional-Medicine Society
http://www.atms.com.au/journal/
English

Reports on the activities of the Australian Traditional Medicine Society and publishes articles related to complementary medicine in Australia. The Web site provides only "instructions to authors" and the tables of contents of issues from 2000 to 2001 and from 2006 to 2007. Users may request a sample copy through e-mail.

Journal of Traditional Chinese Medicine
http://www.jtcm.com
English

Jointly sponsored by the China Association of Traditional Chinese Medicine and Pharmacy and the China Academy of Traditional Chinese Medicine, this journal appeared in 1955 and launched its English edition in 1981. It is published quarterly and devoted to clinical and theoretical research. Its contents include Expert's Forum, Clinical Observation, Basic Investigation, Reviews, Lectures, Teaching Round, and Questions and Answers involving acupuncture, massage therapy, and Chinese *Materia Medica*. The Web site provides the latest information on the development of Traditional Chinese Medicine. Through the Web site, readers can search the tables of contents from 1990 to 2007, keywords, and author names.

Journal of Traditional Chinese Medicine
http://www.jtcm.net.cn
Chinese (simplified)

The Web site is co-sponsored by the China Association of Traditional Chinese Medicine and the China Academy of Traditional Chinese Medicine and is edited and published by the *Journal of Traditional Chinese Medicine* Publishing House. It introduces the history of the journal and provides Chinese-language indexes of issues published between 1998 and 2007.

Journal of Traditional Chinese Medicine
http://www.jtcm.net.cn/include-e.asp
English

The English edition of the *Journal of Traditional Chinese Medicine* aims to provide a platform for exchanging ideas on TCM and disseminating theories on TCM, and demonstrating the development of scientific and technological results on TCM. The English edition of the journal is a quarterly devoted to research on Chinese medicine, both clinically and theoretically. Main columns include Experts' Forum, Clinical Observation, Basic Investigation, Reviews, Lectures, Teaching Round, Acupoint Exploration, and Questions and Answers involving acupuncture, massage therapy, and Chinese *Materia Medica*. Papers written by experts in various fields offer the latest information on developments in TCM. The English edition of the *Journal of Traditional Chinese Medicine* contains valuable references for clinical practitioners and other interested parties. Its Web site provides the index of issues published from 1999 to 2003 and in 2006. The English edition of the *Journal of Traditional Chinese Medicine,* despite sharing the same name and the same publisher with its Chinese counterpart, has different contents. The content of the Chinese edition is comparatively more detailed. The journal is also published in several European languages, including German, French, and Italian.

Journal of Traditional Chinese Medicine
http://www.mtc.es/es/
Spanish

Published by Fundación Europea de Medicina Tradicional China, based in Spain. Access to the Web site is only available to subscribers.

North American Journal of Oriental Medicine
http://members.shaw.ca/najom/Credit.htm
English

Traditional Japanese medicine is an integration of the developments in and interpretations of Oriental medicine in Japan. This journal aims to promote the theories and practices of traditional Japanese medicine, including Japanese acupuncture and moxibustion, kampo (herbology), shiatsu, and anma. Although it focuses on Japanese traditional medicine, its contents also cover acupuncture and moxibustion. The Web site does not provide any index or sample issue.

Oriental Medicine
http://www.omjournal.com
English

The purpose of this journal is to provide information on and the education and possible applications of Oriental medicine such as acupuncture, bodywork, herbology, food therapy, Qigong, and other energetic practices. The Web site provides the indexes of all issues published from 1992 to 2006. Free sample issues are available to download.

Oriental Medicine
http://www.pacificcollege.edu/publications/index.html
English

This is a newspaper published by the Pacific College of Oriental Medicine and features in-depth articles on Oriental medicine written by the faculty of the college and other scholars. Entries are mainly short articles. Two issues are published annually. Issues published from 1998 to 2007 can be read in full online.

Pacific Journal of Oriental Medicine
https://www.cinahl.com/cgi-bin/jrlshowtitles?pjom
English

The Web site lists only the indexes of volumes 14 (1999) to 21(2001).

The European Journal of Integrated Eastern and Western
Medicine
http://www.euro-tcm.org/journal.html
English

As an official journal of Euro-TCM, this journal publishes articles on topics covering clinical TCM, the integration of Eastern and Western medicine, acupuncture, meridians, *Compendium of Materia Medica,* TCM education, Tuina, Qigong, and Taiji Quan. One of the most important sections of the site displays abstracts of scientific papers that have been published in famous journals of Chinese medicine in Mainland China, such as the *Beijing Journal of Traditional Chinese Medicine,* the *Shanghai Journal of Acupuncture and Moxibustion, Acupuncture Research,* the *Journal of Traditional Chinese Medicine, Chinese Acupuncture Moxibustion,* and the *Chinese Journal of Traditional and Western Medicine.* Its Web site does not provide full-text articles or tables of contents. The sample issue is not available for download.

The International Chinese Medical Journal of Daytona
http://chinesetherapeutics.org/journalhome.html
English

The International Chinese Medical Journal of Daytona aims to provide useful information for understanding, applying, integrating, and benefiting from Chinese Medical therapeutics as well as other natural medicines and practices, for both individual and global medical needs. The Web site contains only an introduction and provides little information.

The Lantern: A Journal of Traditional Chinese Medicine
http://www.thelantern.com.au/
English

For students and practitioners, this journal offers useful articles and case studies on Chinese medicine, including acupuncture, herbal medicine, Qigong, Tuina, herb cultivation, or other modalities. The Web site provides only indexes of each issue published from 2004 to 2007.

The TCM Journal
http://the_tcm_journal.tripod.com/
English

TCM Journal is a free online monthly journal. Simply by providing an e-mail address, users can automatically receive the newsletter from the journal free of charge. Most entries on the Web site are short articles, and there are introductions on basic Chinese medical concepts. There is no author guide on the Web site, and there is no evidence that articles are peer-reviewed.

ACUPUNCTURE

Acupuncture and Electro-Therapeutics Research, The
   International Journal
http://www.cognizantcommunication.com/
English

The mission of this journal is to provide a forum for the exchange of ideas and the promotion of basic and clinical research in acupuncture, electro-therapeutics, and related fields. According to the journal's Web site, it also aims to make acupuncture and electro-therapeutics a universally acceptable branch of medicine through multidisciplinary research based on scientific disciplines. Its ultimate goal is to provide a better understanding of both the beneficial and adverse effects of these treatments, to supplement and improve existing methods of diagnosis, prognosis, treatment, and prevention of diseases in both Western and Oriental medicine. The Web site provides indexes of issues printed from 1998 to 2006 with English abstracts and an author index.

Acupuncture in Medicine
www.acupunctureinmedicine.org.uk
English

Published by the British Medical Acupuncture Society, *Acupuncture in Medicine* is a scientific and clinical journal targeting Western-trained physicians and other health professionals. It uses the prevailing theories in neurophysiology and anatomy to interpret the effects of acupuncture. The journal largely restricts its published articles to this Western approach. It publishes scientific reports, systematic and general reviews, audits, case reports, etc., related to medical acupuncture and related techniques from various aspects such as clinical, experimental, technical, and basic science. Summaries of articles printed in previous issues of the journal are available on its Web site free of charge, along with the full text of selected articles.

Acupuncture Today
http://www.acupuncturetoday.com/
English

Acupuncture Today is a monthly online journal. It publishes news, original articles, case reports, and other items of relevance to the acupuncture and Oriental medicine profession.

Akupunktur & Traditionelle Chinesische Medizin
http://www.mlverlag.de/texte/textseite_zeit_aku.htm
German

Publishes articles on acupuncture and Chinese medicine in Germany. Its Web site offers the tables of contents from 1999 to 2004. It is uncertain where the journal is still being published.

American Journal of Acupuncture
http://acupuncturejournal.com/
English

The Web site was established for the *American Journal of Acupuncture,* but the journal is no longer being published. The Web site only provides the contents of journals from 1979 to 1999 as well as three sample articles. The Web site gives an introduction to the journal, which was delivered to AAOM members only.

Chinese Acupuncture and Moxibustion
http://www.cintcm.com/magazine/Acupuncture/index.htm
http://www.cjacupuncture.com/
English

This Web site is affiliated with a journal on Chinese acupuncture and moxibustion. It provides information about Chinese acupuncture. Contents of journals from 2001 to 2007 are available online.

Clinical Acupuncture & Oriental Medicine
http://intl.elsevierhealth.com/journals/caom/default.cfm
http://www.harcourt-international.com/journals/caom
English

The mission of this journal is to provide clinical information, including original research, research reviews, organization reports, educational issues, the management of clinical problems, and international news for the practitioners of acupuncture and interested parties. The journal has ceased to be published.

International Journal of Clinical Acupuncture
http://www.allertonpress.com/journals/acup.htm
English

> In order to serve as a source for introducing to the world a variety of articles reporting the latest developments in clinical acupuncture research, this journal aims to provide a platform for improving practitioners' clinical skills and helping to integrate acupuncture into conventional medical practice. It publishes articles related to acupuncture theory and mechanism research, which are mainly from China, and reports on diseases that are commonly seen in Western acupuncture practice. The Web site is an introductory to the journal and provides only the tables of contents of the latest issue. A sample copy is provided by the publisher upon request.

Japanese Acupuncture and Moxibustion
http://www.jsam.jp/english/journal/index4.php
English and Japanese

> This is an online English journal of the Society of Acupuncture and Moxibustion. The journal mainly publishes original research and case reports related to acupuncture and moxibustion. The Web site offers 2004-2006 issues free of charge.

Journal of the Chinese Medical Association of Acupuncture
http://www.cmaa.org.tw/acup.htm
Chinese (traditional)

> Publishes articles on acupuncture, including the history of acupuncture. Full-text articles published between 1999 and 2003 are available free of charge.

Journal of the Japan Society of Acupuncture and Moxibustion
http://www.jsam.jp/english/index_03.htm
English and Japanese

Published by the Japan Society of Acupuncture and Moxibustion, this journal mainly publishes original research and case reports. Its Web site provides English and Japanese abstracts from 2001 to 2006 with a retrieval system. Sample articles are available on the Web site.

Medical Acupuncture: A Journal for Physicians by Physicians
http://www.medicalacupuncture.org/aama_marf/journal/
  index.html
English

Published by the American Academy of Medical Acupuncture, *Medical Acupuncture* is an online journal focusing on medical acupuncture. It publishes articles on all aspects, including research, education, clinical practice, technology, policy, ethics, law, schools of thought, history, and related disciplines. Full-text articles can be viewed online.

Méridiens
http://www.meridiens.org/m112/entre114.html
French

The Web site contains information about the journal, which is published by Française de Médecine Traditionnelle Chinoise, including its tables of contents from 2002 to 2004. Selected articles can be read online.

Shanghai Journal of Acupuncture and Moxibustion
http://www.tcm-w.com.cn/en/magazine.asp
Chinese (simplified) and English

The Web site only introduces the journal. Users can read articles upon registering.

The Web-Journal of Acupuncture
http://users.med.auth.gr/~karanik/english/webjour.htm
English

The Medical School at the Aristotle University of Thessaloniki in Greece publishes this online journal to offer a platform for school members to share their knowledge and experiences with interested parties. It is updated regularly and provides over a hundred articles. The journal is not peer reviewed. The site provides many links to databases, Web sites on veterinary acupuncture, and e-mail subscriptions.

World Journal of Acupuncture and Moxibustion
http://www.ontcm.com/wjam/index.htm
http://www.ilib.cn/I-sjzjzz-e.2007.02.html
English

Medboo Health Center established this Web site for the online version of the *World Journal of Acupuncture-Moxibustion*. As the official publication of the World Federation of Acupuncture-Moxibustion Societies, it aims to meet the demands of medical professionals and practitioners of TCM for more materials related to all aspects of acupuncture and moxibustion. However, its Web site does not provide further information.

HERBAL

Australian Journal of Medical Herbalism
http://www.nhaa.org.au/index.htm
English

This quarterly journal publishes material on all aspects of medical herbalism, covering topics such as philosophy, phytochemistry, pharmacology, and clinical applications of medicinal plants. It is published by the National Herbalists Association of Australia. Sample issues are available on the Web site.

Canadian Journal of Herbalism
http://www.herbalists.on.ca/journal.html
English

Offers informative articles, case studies, and book reviews on current research into herbal medicine. The target audience comprises practitioners, students, and supporters of the uses of medicinal plants. It is published by the Ontario Herbalists Association. When the author browsed the Web site, it provided two free articles, the tables of contents of past issues published from 1992 to 2006, and the latest issue.

Chinese Traditional and Herbal Drugs
http://www.instrument.com.cn/journal/magazine/about.asp/
  strYear/2006/ID/204
Chinese (simplified)

Jointly published by the Tianjin Institute of Pharmaceutical Research and the Chinese Pharmaceutical Association, this journal mainly publishes essays related to the chemical composition, product quality, examination methods, and sources of herbal drugs from chemical and pharmacological perspectives. Other columns include a forum for discussing the modernization of TCM, summaries, short essays, new products, an introduction to the group, academic activities, and other information. The tables of contents of 2004-2007 issues are available on the Web site.

Herbalgram
http://www.herbalgram.org/herbalgram/
http://www.herbalgram.org/bodywise/herbalgram/default.asp
English

Published by The American Botanical Council. This focuses on herb and medical plant research, regulatory issues, market conditions, native plant conservation, and other general aspects of herb use. Users can subscribe to the journal via the Web site.

The site also lists contents of issues dating back to 1990. Users can also order printed copies by filling in an order form.

Journal of Ethnopharmacology
http://www.elsevier.com/wps/find/journaldescription.cws_
  home/506035/description#description
English

According to the journal's Web site, it publishes original articles concerned with the observation and experimental investigation of the biological activities of plant and animal substances used in the traditional medicine of past and present cultures; at the same time, it is dedicated to the exchange of information and opinions about the use of plants, fungi, animals, microorganisms, and minerals and their biological and pharmacological effects based on the principles established through international conventions. This is the official journal of the International Society for Ethnopharmacology (http://www.ethnopharmacology. org), whose studies take an interdisciplinary approach. The site provides online abstracts, tables of contents, and sample issues.

Journal of Herbs, Spices, & Medicinal Plants
http://www.haworthpress.com/web/JHSMP/
English

This refereed and peer-reviewed journal publishes material related to the production, marketing, and utilization of these plants and associated extracts, and makes relevant and efficient information accessible online. The site provides tables of contents and a sample issue.

Medical Herbalism: A Journal for the Clinical Practitioner
http://medherb.com/MHHOME.SHTML
English

Aims to support the herbal practitioner, to preserve and develop the science and art of herbal medicine, and to promote the communication and sharing of clinical methods and experiences. The Web site currently contains the full text of most articles printed in Medical Herbalism in its first eleven volumes (1989 through 2000) and provides sample issues. It appears that the Web site has not been recently updated.

Natural Pharmacy
http://www.liebertpub.com/publication.aspx?pub_id = 47
English

As the official journal of the Society of Natural Pharmacy, this aims to provide pharmacists with information on vitamins and supplements, botanical and herbal medicines, homeopathic preparations, and natural personal care products. The Web site provides only general information on the journal.

QIGONG AND RELATED SITES

Advances in Mind-Body Medicine
http://www.advancesjournal.com/adv
English

Explores the relationships between mind, body, spirit, and health. Selected articles can be viewed online free of charge, and the table of contents of the current issue is available. However, the "current issue" was published in 2004, and the Web site has not been updated since then. The "current issue" posted on the Web site was the winter 2004 issue. The Web site has not been recently updated.

American Journal of Qigong
http://www.nqa.org/journal.html
English

This site explores the many forms of Qigong: movement and stillness, healing and cultivation, growth and change, the dance and the discipline, and the artistry and the science. Its potential audience is American professionals, teachers, students, and practitioners, who are interested in Qigong. It is published by The National Qigong Association. The Web site does not provide any information regarding the journal, except for "Calls for papers."

Journal of Shiatsu and Oriental Body Therapy
http://www.seed.org/jsobt.html
English

Publishes articles and research in this field.

Qi: The Journal of Traditional Eastern Health and Fitness
http://www.qi-journal.com
English

This quarterly journal has published articles on such topics as acupuncture, acupressure, TCM, herbology, Qigong, Taiji quan, therapeutic massage, feng shui, meditation, and Chinese culture since 1991. A sample issue and the tables of contents of issues published between 1991 and 2006 are available on its Web site.

The Web site also provides TCM-related news.

Tai Chi Magazine
http://www.tai-chi.com
English

This is targeted at those interested in Taiji quan, Qigong, and other internal martial arts. The Web site provides indexes of issues from 1997 to 2007.

The journal does not publish academic essays.

Taiji quan and Qigong Journal
http://www.tqj.de/
English

Publishes essays on Taiji quan and Qgong in German, but the Web site provides English abstracts of all articles.

Taijiquan Journal
http://www.taijiquanjournal.com/
English

This site focuses on the ancient art of Taiji quan and is targeted at students, teachers, scholars, and other interested people. The tables of contents are available online.

The "current issue" posted on the Web site was published in 2004. The Web site has not been recently updated.

The Journal of Bodywork and Movement Therapies
http://intl.elsevierhealth.com/journals/jbmt/
English

This site publishes illustrated articles on a wide range of subjects related to everyday clinical practice in private, community, and primary health care settings. *Bodywork and Movement Therapies* includes Taiji and Qigong. It offers readers the latest therapeutic techniques and current professional debates. It also provides essential reading for all those involved in the assessment, diagnosis, treatment, and rehabilitation of musculoskeletal dysfunction. A sample article on Taiji and Qigong is available on the Web site.

CAM JOURNALS

Alternative and Complementary Therapies
http://www.liebertpub.com/publication.aspx?pub_id = 3
English

Offers the latest information on the evaluation of alternative therapies and their integration into clinical practice. It publishes articles on all aspects of alternative medicine, including acupuncture, Chinese medicine, traditional medicine, bodywork, and massage therapies. The Web site provides tables of contents and a free sample issue.

Alternative Medicine
http://www.alternativemedicine.com/
English

This magazine provides the latest news on herbs and supplements, natural beauty products, eating well, and natural household products—plus up-to-date research in the fields of complementary medicine and alternative therapies—to help readers to make informed decisions on purchasing natural products and health care services. The Web site does not provide any information on the journal.

The journal reports on but does not publish research essays.

Alternative Medicine Review
http://www.thorne.com/index/mod/amr/a/amr
English

This peer-reviewed journal, provided by Thorne Research, publishes literature reviews, original research, editorial comments, monographs, and book reviews related to alternative medicine. Thorne Research's customers can access the journal free of charge. Back issues (1996-2006) may also be downloaded free of charge.

Alternative Therapies in Health and Medicine
http://www.alternative-therapies.com/at
English

This site aims to provide a forum for sharing information on the practical use of alternative therapies in preventing and treating disease, healing illness, and promoting health. According to the Web site, it publishes a variety of disciplined inquiry methods, promotes the evaluation and appropriate use of all effective approaches from the physical to the transpersonal, and encourages the integration of alternative therapies with conventional medical practices in a way that provides for a rational, individualized, comprehensive approach to health care. It publishes articles, brief reports, and article reviews that cover the following topics: acupuncture, Tibetan medicine, Traditional Chinese Medicine, Qigong, massage, and five-element Chinese medicine. The Web site provides only the tables of contents for current and past issues.

BMC Complementary and Alternative Medicine
http://www.biomedcentral.com/1472-6882
English

This site aims to publish original research articles on complementary and alternative health care interventions, with an emphasis on those explaining biological mechanisms of action. Articles published can be accessed online by all. The Web site also has a "Quick Search" function.

Complementary Therapies in Clinical Practice
http://intl.elsevierhealth.com/journals/ctnm/
English

Formerly named *Complementary Therapies in Nursing & Midwifery,* this is a refereed journal that publishes articles to meet the broad-range needs of the health care profession in the effective and professional integration of complementary therapies within clinical practice. According to the journal's Web site, the journal, promoting safe and efficacious clinical practice, publishes rigorous peer-reviewed papers addressing research, the implementation of Complementary and Integrative medicine in the clinical setting, legal and ethical concerns, evaluative accounts of therapy in practice, philosophical analyses of emergent social trends in Complementary and Integrative medicine, excellence in clinical judgment, best practice, problem management, therapy information, policy developments, and the management of change. It is affiliated with the Research Council for Complementary Medicine's CAMRN Network. The Web site provides tables of contents and a free sample issue.

Complementary Therapies in Medicine
http://www.harcourt-international.com/journals/ctim/
English

Affiliated with the Research Council for Complementary Medicine's CAMRN Network, this journal aims to publish research and discussion articles with the main purpose of improving health care. It also provides information and guidance within the field of complementary therapies and publishes a variety of articles including primary research, reviews, and opinion pieces. It has an abstracts section with details of recently published research, as well as information and experiences on integrating complementary medicine into mainstream care. The Web site offers tables of contents and a free sample issue.

Evidence-based Complementary and Alternative Medicine
http://ecam.oxfordjournals.org/
English

This international and peer-reviewed journal seeks to understand sources and to encourage rigorous research in complementary and alternative medicine. The journal publishes articles on basic and clinical research, methodology, and history and the philosophy of medicine related to Traditional Chinese

Medicine and Kampo medicine. It is available in both a printed version and an online version. All papers published in the journal can be obtained online free of charge.

Evidence-Based Integrative Medicine
http://www.medscape.com/viewpublication/1048_index
English

This journal focuses on an evidential basis for incorporating complementary or alternative health care practices with conventional medical approaches, to form a model of health care centered on overall wellness. The Web site provides only the titles of volume 1 No.1 (Chinese Medicine and Supportive Cancer Care) and volume 1. No. 2. Whether this journal is still being published is not known.

Explore: The Journal of Science and Healing
http://ees.elsevier.com/explore/
English

Focuses on the scientific principles behind, and applications of, evidence-based healing practices from a wide variety of sources, including conventional, alternative, and cross-cultural medicine. It is an interdisciplinary journal that explores the healing arts, consciousness, spirituality, eco-environmental issues, and basic science, as all these fields relate to health. The Web site provides tables of contents, abstracts, and a sample issue.

Focus on Alternative and Complementary Therapies
http://journals.medicinescomplete.com/journals/fact/current/
English

Published by the Department of Complementary Medicine, University of Exeter, U.K., this quarterly journal aims to present evidence on complementary and alternative medicine in an analytical and impartial manner. It systematically searches the world literature to uncover articles on CAM research and provides a comprehensive overview of new research, as well as structured summaries and critical appraisals of the most important factual papers. It publishes interviews, debates, summaries, short reports, news, book reviews, and lists of new books and recent literature. The contents of the journal are also listed. Selected items and a sample issue can be viewed online.

Forschende Komplementarmedizin und Klassische Naturheilkunde (Research in Complementary and Classical Natural Medicine)
http://content.karger.com/ProdukteDB/produkte.asp?Aktion = JournalHome&ProduktNr = 224242#english
English and German

This peer-reviewed journal publishes articles in German or English on basic and practice-related research, clinical studies, methodology, and scientific theory in complementary medicine. Tables of contents, abstracts, and sample issues are available on the Web site. All columns, such as "Letters to the Editor," "Documentation," and "Book Reviews" are available free of charge online, except for "Original Articles," for which only abstracts are available free of charge.

Health and Healing: Journal of Complementary Medicine
http://www.healthandhealing.com.au/
English

The Web site provides only the tables of contents. The journal mainly reports on complementary medicine and does not publish research essays.

Integrative Medicine Insights
http://la-press.com/journals.php?pa = toc&journal_id = 21
English

An open-access research journal, it publishes original research papers, short communications, application notes, reviews, case studies, and letters related to the application of complementary and alternative medicine. This is a new journal that is not yet in publication.

Internet Journal of Alternative Medicine
http://www.ispub.com/ostia/index.php?xmlFilePath = journals/ ijam/front.xml
English

This is an open-access journal in which articles, case reports, and press releases can be found. There are five issues to date, and there are several research essays on the topic of acupuncture.

International Journal of Naturopathic Medicine
http://www.intjnm.org/
English

This is a multidisciplinary and Internet-delivered journal that aims to publish research into complementary and alternative medicines, including but not limited to mind-body medicine, acupuncture, allopathic medicine, Asian medicine, botanical medicine, chiropractic/manipulation, clinical nutrition, counseling, hydrotherapy, and massage/physical medicine. Tables of contents and abstracts from the current and some selected past issues are available online.

Japanese Journal of Complementary and Alternative Medicine
http://www.jstage.jst.go.jp/browse/jcam
English and Japanese

Published by the Japan Society for Complementary and Alternative Medicine, this journal has open access. It publishes articles and reviews in Japanese with English abstracts, which can be downloaded free of charge.

Journal of Accord Integrative Medicine
http://www.accordinstitute.org/
English

The purpose of this journal is to integrate Chinese medicine (including acupuncture and Qigong), parapsychology, and Western medicine with scientific theories, technologies, and methods. The journal is online and bi-monthly. All papers can be downloaded free of charge. As observed in past issues, it publishes limited essays and mainly publishes the research of the editor-in-chief.

Journal of Alternative and Complementary Medicine
http://www.liebertpub.com/publication.aspx?pub_id = 26
English

Published bimonthly, it includes reports, ideas, commentary, and opinions on therapies currently thought to be outside the realm of conventional Western biomedicine. It includes current concepts in clinical care that will be useful for those who are seeking to evaluate and integrate these therapies into patient-care protocols. A free sample issue can be viewed on the Web site. It is also the official journal of the Society for Acupuncture Research (http://www.acupunctureresearch.org).

Journal of Chinese Integrative Medicine
http://www.jcimjournal.com/en/index.aspx
English and Chinese

This is an open-access journal. The Web site provides the issues from 2003 to 2007.

Journal of Complementary and Integrative Medicine
http://www.bepress.com/jcim/
English

This journal publishes significant research focusing on evidence concerning the efficacy and safety of complementary and alternative medical whole systems, practices, interventions, and natural health products, including herbal medicines and their integration with allopathic/orthodox medicine. It publishes reviews, research papers, case reports, discussion papers, short notes, conference presentations, proceedings, and noncommercial and commercial advertising. The Web site also provides news from the Canadian Institute of Chinese Medicinal Research.

Journal of Complementary Medicine
http://www.jnlcompmed.com.au/
English

This journal is dedicated to bring evidence-based complementary medicine to the mainstream primary health care provider. It informs the conventional practitioners of treatments used by their patients, to explain the evidence behind them, and to educate the practitioners on how to expand their current practice to integrate those holistic treatments, which are desired by increasing numbers of patients. The journal contents are listed online, and selected articles can be downloaded free of charge.

Seminars in Integrative Medicine
http://www.elsevier.com/wps/find/journaldescription.cws_
  home/623246/description#
English

This provides a forum for discussing the growing field of integrative medicine, in which the journal examines alternative approaches to treatment in a variety of specialties and how they can be integrated with more traditional therapies. The Web site provides tables of contents and a free sample issue.

Seminars in Preventive and Alternative Medicine
http://us.elsevierhealth.com/product.jsp?isbn = 15564061
English

This provides resources for the latest evidence on the use of alternative medicine in the prevention and treatment of chronic diseases, including cancer. Each quarterly issue offers analyses of alternative measures for both the prevention and treatment of chronic diseases, including comparisons of the efficacy of alternative versus traditional treatment. The journal also presents information based on reports from clinical trials to provide guidance in developing individualized patient health plans. It publishes reviews of treatment options and preventive measures from leaders in the field, results of clinical trials, examinations of the benefits and limitations of new products or screening tests, updates on nutritional therapies, supplements, and diets. The Web site provides tables of contents and a free sample issue.

The Australian Journal of Holistic Nursing
http://www.scu.edu.au/schools/nhcp/ajohn/
English

A twice-yearly journal, includes news items, discussions and debates, and documents the dynamic trends in contemporary holistic practice. It includes articles on the practice of natural therapies and holistic nursing. The journal is published by the School of Nursing and Health Care Practices, Southern Cross University, in association with the Australian College of Holistic Nurses, Inc. However, it ceased publication in October 2005. Readers may search the contents by topics or by issue. The Web site provides tables of contents along with abstracts. In "Acupuncture and Traditional Chinese Medicine" users can search for relevant essays and book reviews.

The Scientific Review of Alternative Medicine
http://www.sram.org
http://www.quackwatch.org/04ConsumerEducation/sram.html
English

According to the journal's description, the purpose of this journal is to apply the best tools of science and reason to determine whether hypotheses are valid and treatments are effective. The Web site posts tables of the contents along with abstracts from the current issue and some back issues. Selected articles can be viewed online. The Web site also highlights the latest news on alternative medicine from the Commission for Scientific Medicine and Mental Health.

NEWSLETTERS

Access
http://www.nhaa.org.au/index.htm
English

Access is the quarterly newsletter of the National Herbalists Association of Australia. It aims to keep association members up to date on the activities of the board, as well as on events and industry trends. There is little information on the Web site.

Acubriefs Newsletter
http://www.acubriefs.com/newsletters/newsletter_08.03.htm
English

Maintained by the Medical Acupuncture Research Foundation, the Web site only shows newsletters published between 2000 and 2003. *Acubriefs Newsletter* lists its three objectives: To provide a centralized resource for reviewing new citations on acupuncture in English; to provide annotated abstracts on citations of particular interest to clinicians and researchers; and to facilitate access to citations quoted/reviewed. The Web site also collects free articles and abstracts about Chinese medicine and acupuncture from the Internet, mainly PubMed. It has not been updated for some time.

Alternative Health News Online
http://www.altmedicine.com/
English

This newsletter aims to offer complementary and preventive health news pages on the Internet. The Web site can be searched using the term "Alternative Health News on the Internet," and it attempts to provide some of the "most informative and credible sites." However, the Web sites listed carry little scientific evidence. The published contents are categorized into "What's New," "E-Mail Newsletter," "Health News Bulletins," "Search," "Diet and Nutrition," "Mind/Body Control," "Alternative Medical System," "Manual Healing," and "Health News." It provides the abstracts of up-to-date research achievements. Some abstracts are put on the Web site, and some are linked to PubMed.

Alternative Medicine Alert
http://www.ahcpub.com/archive/?efrlk = 162
http://www.altmednet.com/titles/ama.html
English

This site aims to provide clinically sound information on alternative medicine for medical professionals. This newsletter lists its objectives: present evidence-based clinical analyses of commonly used alternative therapies; make informed, evidence-based recommendations to clinicians about whether to consider using such therapies in practice; and describe and critique the objectives, methods, results, and conclusions of useful, current, peer-reviewed clinical studies in alternative medicine as published in the scientific literature. *Alternative Medicine Alert* is a twelve-page monthly newsletter. The 2006 index page is available for free download. The contents can be viewed only by subscribers. According to the index of the 2005 issue, there are some articles regarding acupuncture and Taiji.

Alternative Therapies in Women's Health
http://www.ahcpub.com/products_and_services/?prid =
358&spcid = 0,1,12&mtyid = 5&cetid = 0,1,2&pdr =
1&clntr = 0&clntru = /clinical_trials/?clu = 358&mtid = c
English

Published by Thomson American Health Consultants, *Alternative Therapies in Women's Health* is the publication of clinically relevant, objective sources of research and assessment about herbs, dietary supplements, and alternative techniques and modalities for women. This newsletter provides practitioners with unbiased scientific information, practical clinical skills, and tips on how best to counsel patients. It takes a critical look at the effectiveness of alternative therapies for women's health problems and potential uses within conventional medical practice, and analyzes the latest scientific research regarding botanicals and complementary therapies. *Alternative Therapies in Women's Health* is an eight-page monthly newsletter. The 2006 index page is available for free download. The contents can be viewed only by subscribers.

According to the index of the 2005 issue, there are some articles regarding acupuncture and Taiji.

China News on Traditional Chinese Medicine
http://www.cntcm.com.cn/
Chinese (simplified)

Provides news about Chinese medicine, how to treat diseases, and famous doctors' formulae.

Chinese Herbal Pharmacy Newsletter
http://www.nesa.edu/pharmacy.html
English

Published by the New England School of Acupuncture. Most articles are short, but users can download them free of charge. The Web site provides, by download, the *Practitioner Guidebook* and *Feb 2005 Newsletter.*

Chinese Medicine Times
http://www.chinesemedicinetimes.com/
English

With six issues a year, this journal is for health care practitioners, students, and those wishing to learn more about the knowledge of Chinese medicine. It is delivered free to Chinese medicine practitioners worldwide, and is an online journal, first published in February 2006. The Web site also selects abstracts of the latest Chinese medical research achievements from other academic journals.

CMA at NIH: Focus on Complementary and Alternative
 Medicine
http://nccam.nih.gov/news/newsletter/2006_winter/
English

Published by the National Center for Complementary and Alternative Medicine (four times a year), this newsletter contains three columns: features, news, and updates to introduce CAM therapies. The current issue and back issues are all available online.

The Web site lists sources and references relevant to its articles, making the Web site very practical. The Web site contents are easy to understand, and it frequently reminds visitors how to use CAM treatment safely.

Guidepoints: Acupuncture in Recovery
http://acudetox.com/index.php?page_name =
  about#guidepoints
English

Guidepoints is the official member newsletter published by the
National Acupuncture Detoxification Association and is only
delivered to members or subscribers. The journal is a health
care-field publication devoted to the subject area of acupunc-
ture-based treatment of addictions and related disorders. The
Web site provides little information.

Jing-Luo
http://www.acupuncture.org.au/newsletter.cfm
English

This is a quarterly newsletter, published by the Australian Acupuncture and Chinese Medicine Association, for its members.
However, it is also available online free of charge. It reports
only on news regarding the Australian Acupuncture and Chinese Medicine Association.

Herb World News Online
http://www.herbs.org/current/topnews.html
English

Maintained by the Herbal Research Foundation, the Web site
collects the latest news that can be read on the Web. The contents are divided into top news, world news, science news, research reviews, politics, industry, and features. The Web site
has its own search engine and is user-friendly, and the contents
are comprehensive.

It appears that information has not been updated online since
2001.

International Health News
http://vvv.com/HealthNews/
English

International Health News aims to provide online information about the latest research in health, nutrition, and medicine. The newsletter offers concise, understandable, and timely summaries of the most important discoveries, based on reviewing over fifty of the world's most respected medical and scientific journals. It focuses on complementary and preventive medicine (specifically in regard to diet, supplements, vitamins, exercise, and lifestyle), reports on the latest treatments for arthritis, cancer, heart disease, and other degenerative conditions, and reviews medical procedures and side effects of pharmaceutical drugs. The Web site provides archives, which include all essays published since 1999 in full-text. Users can also search past news by subject or keyword in the database provided. The Web site in particular serves as an introduction to Chinese herbal medicine.

Kampo News
http://www.honsousa.com/Research/defult.htm
English

The Web site offers summaries of articles, which are all in PDF format and free to download, but only volumes 1 and 2 are available online.

**National Institute of Complementary Medicine: Newsletter and
  Forum**
http://www.nhaa.org.au/index.htm
English

This is a free newsletter published by the National Herbalists Association of Australia. All issues can be downloaded from the Web.

News Journal of the Japan Society of Acupuncture and Moxibustion
http://www.jsam.jp/english/news/index.htm
English and Japanese

The Web site offers news about the study and development of acupuncture and moxibustion in Japan. Ceased production since 2004.

News on Chinese Medicine
http://www.sinbun.co.jp/kampo/kampo.html
Japanese

An online newsletter that mainly reports news on Traditional Chinese Medicine in Japan. The last update was in September 2005.

Newsletter Council of Colleges of Acupuncture and Oriental Medicine
http://www.ccaom.org/
English

Provides only information on the activities of the council.

Oriental Medicine Monthly Newsletter
http://www.acupuncture-websites.com
English

Delivered through e-mail. There is no concrete information on the Web site.

Points Newsletter
http://www.acupuncture.com/newsletters/index.htm
English

Publishes articles covering topics on all aspects of Traditional Chinese Medicine. It has short articles and a section on "recent research," in which it extracts the latest Chinese medical research from PubMed.

Qigong News Founded by Frances Ann McKenzie
http://www.qigongnews.com/
English

Qigong News, delivered by e-mail free of charge, aims to promote public awareness of the health benefits of Qigong.

Qi-Unity Report
http://www.aaaomonline.org/
English

Published by the American Association of Acupuncture and Oriental Medicine, the latest can be viewed on the Web site.

The Newsletter of The Accreditation Commission for Acupuncture and Oriental Medicine
http://www.acaom.org/newsletter.asp
English

Published by The Accreditation Commission for Acupuncture and Oriental Medicine, issues published between 2003 and 2007 can be downloaded free of charge.

The Accreditation Commission for Acupuncture and Oriental Medicine is a school that provides Chinese medical programs, and the newsletter mainly reports on school-related news.

HISTORY AND PHILOSOPHY

Chinese & International Philosophy of Medicine
http://www.cdnet.edu.cn/mirror/hk_college/hkbu/cae.hkbu
.edu.hk/html/CIPM/c_ipom.html
Chinese (simplified)

Published by the Center for Applied Ethics, Hong Kong Baptist University, the Web site only shows the journal's cover page for issues published between 1998 and 2000. No other information is provided online. The journal mainly publishes essays of medical philosophy and ethical topics.

Chinese Journal of Medical History
http://zhyszz.periodicals.net.cn/default.html
Chinese (simplified)

Jointly published by the Chinese Medical Association and the China Academy of Traditional Chinese Medicine, the *Chinese Journal of Medical History* is very renowned. It specifically publishes articles about Chinese medical history and the latest news. Through the WangFang database, its Web site introduces the journal and lists detailed contents from the last four years. The journal can be searched in English through Medline's U.S. Web site (http://www.ncbi.nlm.nih.gov/Pubmed). Those interested can type in "Zhonghua Yi Shi Za Zhi" or other keywords to search the database. This is the only journal that publishes medical history occurring both inside and outside China. The articles are short, but they reflect the latest research on Chinese medical history in Mainland China. It is an important journal in its field.

East Asian Science, Technology, and Medicine
http://www.uni-tuebingen.de/sinologie/eastm
English

Currently published by the University of Tübingen, Germany, it provides articles and book reviews of the science, technology, and medicine of traditional and contemporary East Asia. It is the official publication of the International Society for the History of East Asian Science, Technology, and Medicine. It also provides information on publications, meetings, seminars, grants, and fellowships. Contents of the latest issue can be found through its Web site.

Although not every issue publishes essays on medical history, the essays published in this journal are of high quality.

Korean Journal of Medical History
http://medhist.kams.or.kr/index_e.html
Korean

Published by the Korean Society for the History of Medicine, this journal mainly publishes essays in Korean, although it provides English abstracts for the convenience of researchers who do not read Korean. The articles published in the *Korean Journal of Medical History* can be readily accessed by all on the Internet.

Journal of the Japan Society of Medical History
http://flcsvr.rc.kyushu-u.ac.jp/~michel/jsmh/journal_j.html
English and Japanese

Mainly publishes articles on Japanese medical history. Although it may seem peculiar to list a Web site about Japanese medical history, nonetheless, traditional Japanese medicine is greatly influenced by Traditional Chinese Medicine: The two have a very close relationship. The journal mainly publishes essays in Japanese, although it provides an English index for the convenience of researchers who do not read Japanese. The Web site also has a "Source Guide: Medical History," where it lists "History of Medicine in Japan: Publications in Western Languages."

The Journal of Classics in East Asian Medicine
http://www.jceam.org/
English

The purpose of this journal is to publish articles related to classical writings of East Asian medicine. The editorial board members include medical professors and historians, who are all researchers of Chinese medicine in the U.S. This is a unique English journal focusing on this field. The Web site only provides the sections of "Welcome" and "Editorial board." The first issue has not yet appeared.

Chapter 6

Databases, Bibliographies, and Electronic Texts

A database is an organized collection of information. Scholars may give it a stricter definition, but for the purposes of this discussion, the author will include a wider spectrum. Web sites that offer organized collections of information related to TCM, CAM, and herbs are included in this chapter. Databases mainly provide several kinds of materials, such as bibliographies, periodicals, and essays in full-text. The collection of information, which requires much time and labor, is never an easy task. In order to sustain their functioning, most databases are commercial unless supported by governmental or nonprofit organizations. It is also indisputable that the improving performance of the Internet has played a role in the growing power of these databases.

In the past decade, TCM databases have grown rapidly.[1] The number of studies on TCM have risen each year and free online TCM databases are growing. These databases have a vast volume of TCM data. Nevertheless, can readers trust these databases as sources for their research? A professor from the University of California, Berkeley, has been using TCM databases to search for materials needed for research.[2] It has also been proved that the techniques of knowledge discovery (or data mining) can be effectively used in TCM databases.[3] There are other articles that discuss the use of databases and online TCM.[4] Apparently, the remaining question is how to use these databases wisely and time effectively.[5]

It is not surprising that many databases of *Materia Medica* are listed as a result of the emergence of genetic pharmaceutical technol-

A Guide to Chinese Medicine on the Internet

ogy and the increasing interest in biochemistry and ethnopharmacology in the past ten years.[6] It should be noted that there are herbal databases sharing similar titles but include very different herbs. In most databases, names of herbs appear in all Chinese, English, and Latin.

There is quite a number of TCM-related software on the Internet. Some provide photos of Chinese herbs, some provide herbal and medical formulae, and some of them are databases of acupuncture points, which list acupoint names, meridians, and points with detailed indications and hints to locate the points. Readers can easily search them through search engines. Mostly the demo version can be downloaded to a PC or PDA for free. Each of the software has different functions, and readers should choose with care. The author has never used or tested the functions of these software modules and suggests that readers try the demo version before purchasing.

DATABASES

Academic Information and Library System for Chinese Medical Science
http://www.wenxian.sdutcm.edu.cn/wx/information/information.htm
Chinese (simplified)

The Web site is developed by the Chinese Documentary Research Institute. It is based on current research on ancient Chinese documents, combined with modern informational technology. The system has functions such as editing, categorizing and saving of articles, and a complete text search and a search by categories.

A Comprehensive Acupuncture Points Database
http://www.acumedico.com/acupoints.htm
English

This online database, created by Shmuel Halevi, aims to enhance the knowledge of acupuncture for practitioners and interested people. Every meridian point is Web linked to its parent meridian sketch on this Web site for quick and easy reference. To ease your navigation between the points, the following is a linkage map to each group of points: Lung, Large intestine, Stomach, Spleen, Heart, Small intestine, Bladder, Kidney, Pericardium, Sanjiao, Gall bladder, Liver, Renmai, Dumai, Extra meridian points. Every acupoint is marked with name, definition, energetics, symptoms, combinations, peculiarities, and colorful illustrations. The Web site also has a forum for users interested in discussing acupuncture or Chinese medicine.

Acubriefs
http://www.acubriefs.com/
English

Acubriefs is a subscription-based site that hosts a database of key publications and reviews about acupuncture. Membership brings access to the entire database, including search capabilities, a newsletter, and an acupuncture manual. The database includes publications and abstracts translated from Chinese into English. Yearly dues are moderate, but the newsletter can be procured for free. Acubriefs is currently edited by James K. Rotchford, MD, MPH, and was funded by grants from the Medical Acupuncture Research Foundation and the Best of Both Worlds Foundation. The Web site provides three databases: (1) References Database: Users can search by keyword, specialty, author, date, or all details for specific results. Here journal articles and reviews are available. (2) Reviews Database: Users can search for reviews in past newsletters published by Acubriefs by keyword, author, date, or all details for specific results. (3) Acupuncture Manual: Users can search the Reference Manual for information regarding a specific topic by entering the keyword in the search bar. Users can use the abbreviation for the meridian followed by a dash to choose a number or Pinyin name for the point. Users can actually search the manual by any word or any combination of words.

Acupoints Database Search System
http://www.lifence.ac.jp/cs/adss/
English

The Acupoints Database Search System is a free service created by the development team of Drs. Y. Takaoka, C. Fukuhara, and A. Sugano in 1999. The Web site offers the ability to browse more than 400 acupoints as well as to search through these using the Japanese or Chinese name, the WHO number, or the source. The information on this Web site is intended for noncommercial purposes only, as it comes from the publication *Acupoints & Meridians—A Complement Work of Present Acupuncture and Moxibustion,* published by Huaxia Publishing House in 1997.

Acupuncture Database
http://www.teach100.com/
http://iam.acutimes.com/show_right.asp?liststate = 0&class = 84
Chinese (simplified)

Created by the Institute of Acupuncture and Moxibustion, China Academy of Chinese Medical Sciences, the Web site contains seven databases: Bibliography of Ancient Acupunctural Texts Resource Database (containing over 700 acupunctural texts), Meridians Database (containing eighty medical texts on acupuncture and meridians), Acupoint Database (containing eighty medical texts on acupoints), Moxibustion Database (containing eighty medical books and ancient texts on moxibustion), Acupuncture treatment Database (containing excerpts on acupuncture treatment from eighty ancient texts), Ancient Doctors Database (includes biographies of 1,800 doctors from ancient times to present), and Acupunctural Instruments Database (divided into ancient part and modern part). The site introduces the contents of these databases.

AMED—Allied and Complementary Medicine Database
http://www.bl.uk/collections/health/amed.html
English

> Created by the British library, AMED is a unique bibliographic database produced by the Health Care Information Service of the British Library. It covers a selection of journals in three separate subject areas: (1) several professions allied to medicine; (2) complementary medicine; (3) palliative care.

The Arthritis and Complementary Medicine Database
The Complementary and Alternative Medicine and Pain
   Database
http://www.campain.umm.edu/Databases.html
http://www.compmed.umm.edu./Databases.html
English

> Supported by the National Center for Complementary and Alternative Medicine, the Center for Integrative Medicine, University of Maryland, has developed, and regularly updates, two bibliographic databases: The Arthritis and Complementary Medicine Database and the Complementary and Alternative Medicine and Pain Database. These databases are compiled from regular, comprehensive electronic and manual searches of scientific literature sources worldwide. The Web site also maintains the Cochrane Complementary Medicine Field Registry of Randomized Controlled Trials. The Web site can be searched by typing in keywords. Access to these databases is free.

Note: News and information updated everyday. Interested people can browse the Web site of Center for Integrative Medicine, University of Maryland (http://www.umm.edu/cim/).

Centralised Information Service for Complementary Medicine
http://www.rccm.org.uk/ciscom/CISCOM_intro.aspx
English

The database, created by the Research Council for Complementary Medicine, collected many citations and abstracts covering all the major complementary therapies. Unfortunately, the council is currently reviewing the CISCOM database, and search service is suspended until the review is completed.

Center for Research and Development on New Drug
http://www.chemdrug.com/
http://www.chemdrug.com
http://www.chemdrug.net
http://www.chemdrug.org
http://www.chemdrug.cn
http://www.chemdrug.com.cn
http://www.chemdrug.net.cn
Chinese (simplified)

Although the center is commercial, it has three free TCM databases online. Quality Standard for Chinese Medicinal (with 798 entries) (http://www.chemdrug.com/Zstands.asp), TCM Herbal Database (with 7,314 entries) (http://www.chemdrug.com/Herbal.asp), and TCM Prescription Database (with 10,704 entries) (http://www.chemdrug.com/Prescription.asp). The entries in the three databases are listed by Pinyin system order. After registration, users can use the pharmaceutical literature search service.

Chinadbs.com
http://www.chinadbs.com/search/index.php
Chinese (simplified)

The Web site provides searches on goods produced in China. "Drugs" is among the categories, which allows users to search with keywords under "Chemical Medicine and Biological Sedative," "Chinese Formulated Prescriptions," "Chinese Medicinal Herbs and Tablets," and "Animal Medicine." Nevertheless, users will have to pay to read the products' details. The Web site also includes two other databases related to Chinese medicine, which are not provided for free: The Database of Formulated Chinese Prescription Products in China (http://www.chinadbs .com/search/ki11815910.html) and The Compendium of Chinese Medicinal Resources in China (http://www.chinadbs.com/ search/ki11465835.html).

China Biomedicine Literature Database
http://cbmwww.imicams.ac.cn/
Chinese (simplified)

Established by the Institute of Medical Information, China, the database collects over 1,600 biomedical journals and 3 million articles. Users can try the database (http://cbm.imicams.ac.cn/ cbmbin/login.dll), according to title, author, abstract, keyword, etc. for free.

China INFOBANK-China Medical and Health
http://www.chinainfobank.com/irisweb/english/homepage.htm
Chinese (simplified) with English introduction

This has health- and medical-related news and information from various Chinese health-related newspapers and magazines in China.
News and information update everyday.

Channels and Meridians Database
http://nricm2.nricm.edu.tw/pages/frame-dbsearch1.php
Chinese (traditional)

The Web site is a tool to search for information about acupoints, channels, and meridians. Any entry about acupoints and its location and indication can be searched by names of channels, names of acupoints, location, indication, application, or dosage.

The database is provided by the National Research Institute of Chinese Medicine in Taiwan, and it can be browsed for free.

Chinese Herb Pharmacopoeia
http://www.yncte.com/yd/index.htm
Chinese (Simplified)

Herbs are categorized by their part as applied in medicine (such as roots, fruits, flowers, and leaves). They can also be searched by herb names. The Web site is set up and provided for free by Window of Yunna Country & Township.

Chinese Herbal Project Database
http://www.zhongyanhui.com/NewsView1.asp?id = 408
Chinese (Simplified)

The Web site is currently under construction and only has a brief description on the project.

Chinese Herbs Dictionary
http://alternativehealing.org/chinese_herbs_dictionary.htm
English

Entries can be searched by the first letter of the herbs' Latin names, the first letter of the herbs' Chinese names, or the amount of strokes of the first traditional character of the herbs' Chinese names. The Web site also provides the following information: "toxicity of some herbs," "side effects of some herbs," "herbs that can be toxic to kidneys," "herb that may cause allergy," and "avoiding herbs and drugs interaction." Every entry includes a picture of the herb, its pharmaceutical name, its Latin botanical name, and pronunciation in Japanese, Korean, and Cantonese; its common name, its distribution, its properties, channels and meridians it enters, its medical functions, its actions and indications, its chemical ingredients, samples of formulae, modern usage, cautions and toxicity.

Chinese Herb System
http://www.china-e.com.cn/en/products/ChineseHerb.htm
Chinese (simplified) and English

Zhongyi cooperated with China Medical Research Institution to develop this full-text searchable Chinese herb system. This system is comprised of over 20,000 entries of Chinese herbs, and each entry includes information such as official name, English name, Latin name, nickname, category, derivation, efficacy, and so forth. Statistics analysis is also available.

Note: The Web site only provides a brief introduction without any demo or free trial. The information provided is rather limited. Those who want to learn more would have to contact Zhongyi Electronic Ltd.

Chinese Medicine Digital Library, Medicine Comprehensive Database, Chinese Medicine Statistics Web
http://www.pharmadl.com/pharmadl/zxzjj/sjk.html
Chinese (simplified)

These three databases are set up by the Shanghai Medical Industrial Research Institute Information Center. The Web site only provides a brief introduction without any demonstration of the database. If users want to know more details, they would have to contact the center.

Chinese Medicine Dictionary
http://51qe.cn/index3003.php
Chinese (simplified)

This column collects more than 2,000 entries of Chinese medical terminology and introductions to famous physicians in both ancient and modern history. All entries are sorted alphabetically by their titles in Pinyin.

China Traditional Chinese Medicine Patent Database
http://211.157.104.69/chineseversion/login/index.asp
http://211.157.104.69/englishversion/login/index.asp
Chinese (simplified) and English

The China TCM Patent Database, established by Patent Data Research & Development Center in 2001, is a subsidiary of the Intellectual Property Publishing House of the State Intellectual Property Office of China. The database contains over 19,000 patent records and 40,000 TCM formulas published from 1985 to present. The database provides information on all aspects of TCM patents including development, synthesis, evaluation, manufacture, and application. The site claims that "the unique, state-of-the art indexing of the database enables professionals to quickly and precisely search for information on new development in TCM R&D fields and monitor activities of their competitors based on enhanced title, abstract and subject indexing." In addition, the Patent Data R&D Center provides an online search service. There are twenty-nine search fields in the database that fall into four categories: bibliographic information, subject index terms, uses/effects, TCM formulas. Rewritten titles and abstracts provide users with more searchable information. For further details, please see Liu Y et al. (2004), "China Traditional Chinese Medicine (TCM) Patent Database," *World Patent Information,* 26(1): 91-96. Recently, the Intellectual Property Publishing House of the State Intellectual Property Office of China also collaborate with Chang Chun-Chinese medicine to establish a new database, named "Chinese Medicine Patent Database" which can be found at http://221.8.30.41/nation3.dll.

Complementary and Alternative Medicine Evidence OnLine
http://www.rccm.org.uk/cameol/Default.aspx
English

The Research Council for Complementary Medicine created this Web site along with the School of Integrated Health at the

University of Westminster in London, England. Their goals are to assess published research in the field of complementary or alternative therapies and to make this information available to students, researchers, practitioners, and the public. The database that was generated out of this collaboration is CAM-EOL—Complementary and Alternative Medicine Evidence OnLine. Although the CAMEOL database is a work in progress, one can browse it based on conditions (such as cancer or stroke), or based on therapies (such as acupuncture and yoga). One can also browse all reviews or perform a basic search to obtain more information. Each entry provides information about methods, results, publications, and conclusions, largely about the effectiveness of various treatments.

Computer Retrieval of Information on Scientific Projects
http://crisp.cit.nih.gov/
English

CRISP (Computer Retrieval of Information on Scientific Projects) is a searchable database of federally funded biomedical research projects conducted at universities, hospitals, and other research institutions. The database, maintained by the Office of Extramural Research at the National Institutes of Health, includes projects funded by the National Institutes of Health, Substance Abuse and Mental Health Services, Health Resources and Services Administration, Food and Drug Administration, Centers for Disease Control and Prevention, Agency for Health Care Research and Quality, and Office of Assistant Secretary of Health. Users, including the public, can use the CRISP interface to search for scientific concepts, emerging trends and techniques, or identify specific projects and/or investigators. The Web site only introduces the database without providing an interface.

CORK Database
http://www.projectcork.org/database_search/
English

> The CORK database includes over 69,000 items on substance abuse. These include journal articles, books, book chapters, and reports. The database is updated quarterly and is targeted at conventional medicine. There are subject headings for alternative and complementary practices, such as acupuncture. Online searches can be conducted, either in a "Basic Search Format" or an "Advanced Format." Documentation is available. Users can search by typing in keywords. The contents include many articles about Traditional Chinese Medicine.

Crane Herb Company
http://www.craneherb.com/productlines/SunTen.html
English

> At the Crane Herb Company's Web site, one can find information about Chinese herbs and herbal formulas. This company is compliant with all Food and Drug Administration and Health Insurance Portability and Accountability Act standards and requires registration at the Web site to access certain links. Crane Herb also offers acupuncture supplies and books, and there are numerous forums for discussion. The Web site can be searched by typing in keywords in Pinyin.

Document Retrieval on Ophthalmology of Chinese Medicine
http://www.china-eyecare.com/dataquery/index.php
Chinese (simplified) and English

> The Web site, as part of the online resources of Eye Hospital of China, Academy of Chinese Medical Sciences provides a database based on the databases of the Institute of Information on Traditional Chinese Medicine; users can search documents of Ophthalmology of Chinese Medicine, both ancient and contemporary. The English version is not as user-friendly.

Formulae Database
http://nricm2.nricm.edu.tw/pages/frame-dbsearch2.php
Chinese (traditional)

Information about formulae can be searched by names, composition, functions, or indications. The database is provided by the National Research institute of Chinese Medicine in Taiwan, and it can be used for free.

Herb Medicine
http://www.herbmed.org/
English

HerbMed is a database of over three dozen herbs commonly used in alternative and complementary medicine. This site offers information about the medicinal uses of herbs. Each herb entry is subdivided into additional subject headings, such as Evidence for Efficacy, Safety Data, and Formula/Blends. Articles in these subheadings are listed with full bibliographic citations, often linked to their entry in the PubMed database. Entries for individual herbs are updated regularly. Although most of the information on this Web site is free, certain herbs require a fee to access the professional version.

This public site provides free access to forty-five herbs.

Users can search for herbs by the first letter of their names. Information is given according to the following categories: Scientific Name, Family Name, Common Name, Evidence for Efficacy, Safety Data, Evidence of Activity, Formulas, Dynamic Updates, Other Information, and History of Records. Users have to pay a fee in order to access records of all herbs.

Herbal Database
http://www.okanogan1.com/natural/lifesci/herbal/herbal.htm
English

The Herbal Database is a basic dictionary of a variety of herbs and other natural products. Each botanical element is listed along with its taxonomic name and classification and ways the plant has been used. Some of the information presented is based on folklore and superstition about plants and the author claims no particular expertise in guiding the reader through this catalogue of herbs. This database is solely for informational purposes and has not been reviewed by professional practitioners.

The Herbal Database includes a glossary of terms, an index, and a reference bibliography. The Web site has a downloadable version in PDF format.

Herbal Database
http://gl.purenaturalhealth.com/herbaldb/index.html
English

Herbs are sorted alphabetically on the Web site. Brief introductions of the herbs are provided.

Herbal Medicine
http://herbal.tradetouch.com/
English

The program includes sections on herbal medicine, the properties and characteristics of more than 290 single herbs, and 200 herbal combination formulas for healing and dietary supplements; allows the user to search articles and herbs, and suggests herbal combinations for both diet and health. Information presented in the program is culled from clinical trials, scientific studies, and historical and oral traditions.

Users need to pay to download the software.

Herbs
http://www.herbal-software.com/
English

Herbs is a multilingual database of over 500 herbs distributed by Zentrum Publishing. It currently includes the ability to search herbs by their name in a variety of languages (such as Chinese, English, and Ayurvedic) or by the afflictions the herbs can aid in curing. The Herbs program includes over 100 photographs and allows the user to customize the database with additional entries.

Users need to pay to download the software.

Herbs Database
http://nricm2.nricm.edu.tw/pages/frame-dbsearch2.php
Chinese (traditional)

Data can be searched by names, ingredients, functions, nature-taste, and channel entry. The database is provided by the National Research Institute of Chinese Medicine in Taiwan, and it can be used for free.

Herbs Dictionary
http://www.100md.com/index/0L/a1/20/Index.htm
Chinese (simplified)

Provided by Baimu Medicine, this online dictionary includes names of drugs in Western and Chinese medicines, their other names, generic names, brand names, English names, Latin names, medical terminology, medical abbreviations, etc. The dictionary can be used for free.

Herbasin Chinese Herb Database
http://www.herbasin.com/herbs.htm
English

The Herbasin database lists over 1,000 herbs by their Latin, Chinese, Pinyin, and English names. Many of these have links to information about the herbs, indications for use, administration and dosage, and photographs. Through the database, Herb Origin, Description, Action, Indication, Referential Advice, Tips, Nature, and Affinity, Main Active Ingredient, Precaution and Storage can be also found.

HolisticOnLine
http://www.holistic-online.com/Herbal-Med/Hol_Herb_
   Directory_Index.htm
English

HolisticOnLine presents an index of herb information that can be browsed based on the scientific name or the common name of the herb. Each entry includes a history of the use of the herb, its medicinal qualities, remedies, dosage, and safety precautions. Some entries include photographs. Additional Web pages on this site include information about herbal remedies, an introduction to herbal medicine, and general articles about herbs. This Web site was developed by International Cyber Business Services, Inc. The content includes herbs' names, biological names, parts used, remedies, dosage and safety. It can be used for free.

HOM-INFORM
http://www.hom-inform.org/
English

The British Homeopathic Library is located in the Glasgow Homeopathic Hospital in Scotland. Although this is a physical library, the Web site offers a searchable database of over 25,000 references dealing with homeopathy from the late nineteenth century to the present day. Searches can be initiated in the online database using title, author, language, or keyword. Becoming a member of the library entitles a person to visit the library as well as to request literature searches by the staff of the library. Accessible and free of charge on the Web site is the ECH Homeopathic Thesaurus.

Users can start searching by entering keywords. TCM contents are also included.

Hua Yu Xin Rui
http://www.hyxr.com.cn/cp-shenghuayi.htm
Chinese (simplified)

The company provides the following databases related to Chinese medicine: Chinese Medicine Application System Treasure-house, Chinese Medical Library in CD-Rom: The Complete Record on Acupuncture. The Web site simply provides an introduction to their contents. Users can purchase these databases from the company, which also distributes other databases provided by TCM Online.

Phytotherapies.org
http://www.phytotherapies.org/
English

Phytotherapies is a Web resource, including editorial content, articles, and an extensive searchable and hyperlinked herbal database on current herbal therapeutics, sponsored by the Australian company Herbworx for the professional herbalist. Access to the Web site requires free registration, but it is updated weekly with cross-referenced information about herbal medicine. The site includes both an herbal database and a list of registered practitioners. The database supports boolean searches, such as herb name and disease, and includes information on indications and properties of herbs.

Pictures of Chinese herbs
http://www.bioon.com/figure/List/List_1397.shtml
Chinese (simplified)

The site lists many pictures of Chinese herbs. The site has also English version but it is very brief.

QiGong and Energy Medicine Database Online
http://www.qigonginstitute.org/html/database.php
English

The Qigong and Energy Medicine Database is a bibliographic database of articles, references, and abstracts available for purchase, either in their entirety or on a per-abstract basis. The database currently includes over 3,900 citations for subjects as varied as Qigong, Taiji, Ayurveda, and homeopathy. The database is searchable, and many references are fully abstracted in English. This specialist database is produced by the QiGong Institute. The Qigong Database provides the only record in English of the vast amount of research on Qigong from China as well from other countries. The database contains reports of therapies that have been tried and claimed to be effective. Although users have to pay for each article, they can search for article titles through the database.

Scientific Databases, Chinese Academy of Science
http://www.sdb.ac.cn/viewdb.jsp?uri = cn.csdb.plant.herb
Chinese (simplified)

With reference to the Chinese national pharmacopoeia, the Web site contains 465 Chinese herbs according to their botanic identities, along with relevant information. The database collects information of botanic classification, categories of plants, their medical nature and flavor, diseases targeted, medical parts, chemical ingredients, etc.

The Web site simply introduces the database. Users will have to pay for registration. Another database, Chinese Botanical Database, is also related to Chinese medicine.

Searchable World Wide Web Multilingual Multiscript Plant Name Database
http://www.plantnames.unimelb.edu.au/Sorting/Frontpage .html
English

This free Web service, sponsored by the University of Melbourne in Australia, is a list of numerous herb names translated into over sixty languages and over twenty alphabets. The Web site also features a bibliography and online resources dealing with herbs and herbal medicine. Through the "Generic List" search provided by the Web site, users can find plants with their Chinese name. The Web site also provides a "note on Chinese language," which gives basic information and states its approach to the language used in the database. It has other articles: "Note on Identifying 'Jiaogan' and 'Lugan'", "Chinese Mandarins" International Cooperative Effort," and "Note on Working Out Chinese Names of European Fruit Cultivars."

Shanghai TCM Data Center
http://temdb.sgst.cn/
Chinese (simplified)

The center created TCM Informatics containing eight TCM databases: TCM Disease Database, TCM Recipe Database, TCM Species Database, TCM Compound Database, TCM Compactivity Database, TCM Expert of Shanghai Database, TCM Doctor Database, and Research on TCM Prevention of Cancer Database. These databases are interconnected and can be searched online for free. The site has also very detailed descriptions on these databases.

TCM Herb Library: Introduction, Theory, Herbal Database
http://www.rmhiherbal.org/ai/pharintro.html
English

> Set up by the Rocky Mountain Herbal Institute, the Traditional
> Chinese Medicine herb database includes information on nearly
> 300 plants, along with definitions, patient symptoms, and herb
> formulas. Free registration allows the user to access a limited
> subset of the TCM database. The database targets both health
> professionals and their clients. The Web site also offers the da-
> tabase in a CD format that includes self-study features (such as
> 291 herb entries plus index of common symptoms, 136 TCM
> syndrome definitions, 254 classical herbal formulas, extensive
> cross-referencing for easy look-up of terminology, and indexing
> of terms) for the student of Chinese herbal sciences. Both the
> full and limited versions of the TCM are searchable in English
> and Chinese Pinyin.

TCM Online Databases
http://www.cintcm.com/e_cintcm/e_news/new/news5.htm
http://www.cintcm.ac.cn
http://www.cintcm.com
Chinese (simplified and traditional) and English

> The Traditional Chinese Medical Database System currently
> includes over twenty different databases that are integrated so
> that a user can enter one search term and obtain results from
> all databases if desired. These databases were created and are
> maintained by the Institute of Information on Traditional Chi-
> nese Medicine at the China Academy of Traditional Chinese
> Medicine. The database system includes a literature analysis
> database, traditional Chinese and Tibetan drug databases, a
> database on Traditional Chinese Medicine news, and a clini-
> cal medicine database. This system, in addition to offering an
> integrated search among some or all of the separate databases,
> also lists results by frequency of use or popularity, and could
> be of great use to medical professionals and others interested

in topics of eastern medicine. Access is granted through user registration. The general site also features a user forum, which is mostly in Chinese. Access to the databases is restricted to registered users, and the Web sites only provide an introduction to contents of the databases and with an operation illustration.

TCM Online Databases

1. *Traditional Chinese Medical Literature Analysis and Retrieval Database (TCMLARS) (Chinese).* This database covers Traditional Chinese Medicine (including Chinese herbal medicines, acupuncture, Qigong, Chinese massage, health promotion, etc.) in literature, particularly journals and other periodicals. The database boasts over 477,000 references from over 800 Chinese journals, and all of the information dates from 1984 or later. The user can search on a variety of field names, such as: subject heading, name of disease or diagnosis, usage and dosage, and keywords in English or Chinese abstracts. A more detailed introduction to this TCMLARS databases is available in English at: forge.fh-potsdam.de/~IFLA/INSPEL/01-3fawe.pdf.

2. *Traditional Chinese Medical Literature Analysis and Retrieval System (English).* Like the TCMLARS database, this one, in English, covers recent literature about Chinese medicine (including Chinese herbal medicines, acupuncture, Qigong, Chinese massage, health promotion, etc.) from journals and periodicals. It includes over 73,000 references in English on topics like acupuncture and herbal medicine. A more detailed introduction to this TCMLARS database is available in English at: forge.fh-potsdam.de/~IFLA/INSPEL/01-3fawe.pdf.

3. *Chinese Herb Medicine Database (TCDBASE) (Chinese).* This database, which holds over 8,500 records, deals with Chinese *Materia Medica* and herbal medicine. Individual records provide information about an herb or mineral used in natural medicine, including references to publications. This information is drawn from a variety of sources, such as the Chinese *Materia Medica* Dictionary. The user can find information such as herb name, uses of herbs, pharmacology, dosage, precautions, and storage.

4. *Chinese Herb Medicine Database (English).* This English-language database currently contains over 500 records about the topic of Chinese *Materia Medica* and herbal medicine. Each record represents an herb, and the database provides information on usage, dosage, precautions, and references.

5. *Database of Tibetan Medicines (Chinese).* Over 500 records on Tibetan medicine are included in this database, drawn from traditional sources such as *Yue Wang Yao Zhen, Si Bu Yi Dian,* Ancestor's Dictation, *Jing Zhu Bencao* as well as contemporary published information. Some information that can be found in this database includes: methods of planting, chemical composition, pharmacology, usage and dosage, and toxicology.

6. *Database of Currently Application of Herbal Medicine Formula.* A demo version of this database about Chinese medicine formulas can be found in Chinese at: http://dbshare.cintcm.com/webdkrh1/xdfj/xdfj.asp. There are plans to put out an English version soon. The database contains over 7,500 prescriptions taken from published sources like Pharmacopoeia of the People's Republic of China and Standards for Herbal Medicine Formula. Formula names can be read in English, Latin, or Chinese Pinyin, and include information about ingredients, efficacy, usage, and toxicology.

7. *Database of Chinese Medical Formula (Chinese).* Another database about Chinese medical formula, this contains 86,000 records of formulas. The information contained in this database, such as history of the formulas, ingredients, dosage, and toxicity, is taken from hundreds of ancient medical books. Coverage: It contains 85,989 records. Each record represents a single formula and provides the cited information. Data are derived from more than 700 ancient medical books.

8. *Database of Chemical Composition from Chinese Herbal Medicine (Chinese).* This database contains over 3,000 chemical compositions taken from a variety of sources such as Pharmacology of Traditional Chinese Medicine. The user can learn the chemical name, English name, and formal name, and detailed information is provided on physical, chemical, and biological properties.

9. *Database of Medical Product (Chinese).* For users who want to know about Chinese medical products, this database has over 7,000

records with information taken directly from the manufacturers. In addition to information about the dosage, efficacy, and retail cost of specific products, the user can find out information about the company that manufactures the product, including information about annual sales, export rights, and quality standards.

10. *Database of State Essential Druggery of China (Chinese).* Each of the 825 records in this database deals with medicines used in healing, with information drawn from both Traditional Chinese Medicine and Western medicine. Standard information includes composition of the medicine, pharmacology, usage, and precautions.

11. *Database of New Drug (Chinese).* New medications are often approved by the State Drug Administration, and this database collects information on them. The database contains over 1,500 records, including information about the institution responsible for the creation of the new drug and patent number, in addition to information about dosage, efficacy, and contraindications.

12. *OTC Database (Chinese).* Over-the-counter medical products are collected in this database, using information from the Chinese government. Over 300 records include information about the drug's English and formal name, usage, efficacy, dosage, and precautions.

13. *Medical News Database (Chinese).* A database of over 60,000 records has been created that collects information from Chinese newspapers. The Medical News Database is searchable based on title, author, date, and keywords.

14. *Clinical Medicine Database (Chinese).* This database represents information on over 4,000 different diseases and maladies, with references to publications on both Western medicine and Traditional Chinese Medicine. Each disease entry includes a wealth of information, such as etiology, morbidity, diagnosis, symptoms, prevention, and treatment methods drawn from Western and Chinese medicine.

15. *Traditional Chinese Medicine Pharmaceutical Industry Database (Chinese).* This site provides useful information about the pharmaceutical industry in China. It provides information on over 7,000 companies that deal with Traditional Chinese Medicine, such as name of the company, contact information, Web site, and economic statistics.

16. *China Hospitals Database (Chinese)*. A database of Chinese hospitals with information on over 12,000 hospitals throughout China. The name and contact details of hospitals can be found here, in addition to statistics on outpatients, departments, and number of beds.

17. *Venomous Chinese Herbs Database Platform*. Demo versions of this database have been posted on the Internet at: http://test .cintcm.com/venomousness/index.html and http://dbshare.cintcm .com/venomousness/. This database will include a list of venomous Chinese herbs, along with information on chemical ingredients of the herbs and the way that venomous herbs work. The goal of this database is to use the information currently known on venomousness to help further the field of Traditional Chinese Medicine.

18. *Chinese Medicine Experiment Database: Chemical Ingredient Inquiry (Chinese)*. A demo version of this database is online at: http://dbshare.cintcm.com/HuaXueShiYan/. This database includes over 15,000 records dealing with the chemical analysis of Chinese prescriptions. This database is free for users to browse.

19. *Chinese Medicine Experiment Data Warehouse (Chinese)*. A demo version of this database is available online at: http://dbshare .cintcm.com/ZhongYaoYaoLi/. This database on Chinese pharmacology has gathered references and articles that touch on the subjects of Chinese pharmacology, clinical pharmacology, and venomousness. All of the information contained in this database is drawn from recently published medical journals. The user can search the database from a variety of fields, and the database produces results generated by count frequency.

20. *Chemical Experiment Warehouse (Chinese)*. This demo database can be found online at: http://dbshare.cintcm.com/HuaXueshiYan/tjcondition.htm. This database provides information on chemical experiments. Search results are sorted based on frequency of appearance.

Note: Detailed Chinese descriptions on databases created by the Institute of Information on Traditional Chinese Medicine, China Academy of Traditional Chinese Medicine, please refer to URL: http://dbshare.cintcm.com/webdkrh1/ or http://www.cintcm.com/lanmu/shujuku/index.htm.

It also provides free but very useful TCM databases (simplified Chinese demo version) which contain:

The Database of Journals from Republican China
http://dbshare .cintcm.com/webdkrh1/mgqk/mgqk.asp

The Database of Ancient Chinese Medical Texts Overseas
http://dbshare.cintcm.com/webdkrh1/hwgj/hwgj_search.asp

The Collection of Clinical TCM Jargons
http://sharelab.cintcm.com/TCMCTOntoEdit/demo/test/
browser.html

TCM Linguistic System
http://sharelab.cintcm.com/TCMLSOntoEdit/demo/test/
browser.html

The Web sites of TCM Online (http://www.cintcm.com/e_cintcm/index.htm) and Geneva Foundation for Medical Education and Research (http://www.gfmer.ch/TMCAM/TNCAM_database_system.htm) also have detailed introduction to the databases in English.

Traditional Chinese & Western Herbal Medicine in Humans & Animals
http://homepage.tinet.ie/~progers/herblink.htm#ppdb
English

The site collects many links to herbal databases with brief descriptions.

Traditional Medicine Database
http://www.dynamicarray.com.au/software4TMD.htm
English

The Traditional Medicine Database (TMD) combines Herb-Base and Nutritional Medicine Database for people interested in herbal and nutritional medicine. The TMD contains information on the medicinal properties of over 200 herbs and publications relevant to herbal supplements, and it allows the user to search for health and diet symptoms and prescribe herbs to counteract these issues. There are sixteen searchable fields such as botanical name, constituents, therapeutic applications, dosage, toxicology etc. The TMD is flexible, allowing the user to create and define new fields and customize the database. All databases from this site have free trial versions available.

This is not a free software. Users can download a free trial before purchase.

TCM Research
http://www.tcmresearch.com/
Chinese (traditional)

The database is divided into two sections. The "Chinese Medicine Database" can be searched by names or categories of the medicine. The "Targeted Symptoms" database can be searched by categories of the illnesses. The Web site provides healing formulae and medicine.

Terminology of TCM
http://www.shen-nong.com/chi/tcm/index.html
Chinese (traditional)

Terminology of TCM can be viewed online.

The Biotech, Medi-tech and Chinese Herbal Medicine Patent
  Information Data Search System
http://biotech.tipo.gov.tw
Chinese (traditional)

The Web site is set up by the Intellectual Property Office in Taiwan. It includes a "Chinese Herbal Medicine Database," which covers information of Chinese medicine patents (including patents in Taiwan, Japan, United States, China, Europe, United Kingdom, Germany, and other parts of the world), a database of plants, a database of botanical natural chemical compounds (this database includes 400 kinds of major medical plants and related research articles and structural formula), an ancient Chinese medical classics database (this database collects 350 ancient classics, which are divided into chapters of herbal prescriptions, clinical medicine, medical classics and life-nourishing, and others), a compound prescription search (provides a search for Chinese prescriptions, Chinese medicine patents and Chinese ancient texts; it further provides drug information like names, nature and flavor, meridian tropism, uses, ingredients, targeted diseases, etc.), a Chinese famous prescription search (this database has collected more than 8,000 prescriptions), a Chinese herbal drugs search, a compound with Chinese herbal component database (this database provides a search for compounds of Chinese herbs and their relevant pharmacological information, including their chemical characteristics, toxicity, pharmacological uses, clinical applications, etc.), and an image and illustration search (this database includes images of plants and herbal medicine). The databases can be used for free.

The Chinese Medicine Information Database Inquiry
http://willow.njnet.edu.cn/gonia_medicine/index.htm
Chinese (simplified)

The database collected information of common illnesses and Chinese medical formulae. It can be used for free.

The Chinese Herbs Information Warehouse
http://www.cnwesthotline.com/west01/zcyc00/zcyc.htm
Chinese (simplified)

The Chinese Herbs Information Warehouse is a database of Chinese herbs established by Huaxi Wuzhou Electronic Trading Center of China. This database comprehensively and systematically collected information of Chinese herbal drugs, their names, manufacturers, and other relevant information.

The Encyclopedia of Chinese Herbal Medicine
http://www.yn.edu.cn/yd/
Chinese (simplified)

Plants are categorized by their parts used in medicine. Chinese medicine information is provided and can be searched by keywords.

The Herbal Database, National Complementary Health Council
http://www.nchc2000.org/
English

The Web site lists detailed descriptions with traditional uses of each herb.

TradiMed
http://www.tradimed.com/
English

The TradiMed database has collected information from both Chinese and Korean medicine, and offers this information on a subscription or pay-as-you-go basis. A typical record will present the taxonomic classification of the herb, along with a picture, and give its Latin, English, and Chinese names. There is information on formulation, constituents (including the molecular structure), and the types of diseases for which the herb can be used. The TradiMed database contains the following sections: Herbal taxonomy, Formulae, Constituents, Symptom/ Disease and Processing. The database provides limited samples for free preview.

Viable-herbal, Co.
http://www.viable-herbal.com/herbdesc/herbdesc.htm
English

This Web page is provided as a historical reference of herbal descriptions, including vitamins, minerals, amino acids, and nutrients. Names of herbs are sorted alphabetically.

Yuan Xing Chinese Medicinal Herb Dictionary
http://download.enet.com.cn/html/030282004040203.html
Chinese (simplified)

The page provides detailed information for approximately 800 kinds of common medicinal herbs used across China, with about 200 illustrations. Users can search entries by names, functions, other names, or other methods. The search can be done by typing only the first letter of the Pinyin name. Also there are hundreds of dietotherapy recipes for family use. Users can download the software and add information freely.

JOURNALS AND ARTICLES

Bandolier
http://www.jr2.ox.ac.uk/bandolier/booth/booths/altmed.html
English

The Web site provides abstracts of research on acupuncture, herbs, and massage. It also published the complete text of *Bandolier Journal* (1994-2005) online for free, in which readers can find many articles on Chinese medicine and acupuncture.

CAM on PubMed
http://www.nlm.nih.gov/nccam/camonpubmed.html
English

National Center for Complementary and Alternative Medicine and the National Library of Medicine (NLM) have partnered to create Complementary and Alternative Medicine, a subset of NLM's PubMed. PubMed provides access to citations from the Medline database and additional life science journals. It also includes links to many full-text articles at journal Web sites and other related Web resources.

China Information Service System on Traditional Chinese Medicine
http://www.cintcm.ac.cn/edata/index-e.htm
Chinese (simplified) and English

This site introduces sixteen journals of Traditional Chinese Medicine and allows searching of their tables of contents. Journals include *Chinese Journal of Information on TCM, Chinese Medical Abstract-TCM Section, International Reference on TCM, Research on TCM Policy, Chinese Journal of Integrated Traditional and Western Medicine, Shanghai Journal of Information on TCM, International Advances on TCM Technology, The Journal of the British Medical Acupuncture Society,* and *Hunan Guiding Journal of TCM Pharmacology.*

China National Knowledge Infrastructure
http://www.cnki.net
Chinese (simplified)

China National Knowledge Infrastructure contains the China Hospital Knowledge Databases, which collect full-text journals on biological medicine written in Chinese. Journals are categorized according to topic. This site provides a (fee-based) service for browsing journal articles published in Mainland China by the Chinese Medical Association, and other journals on Chinese medicine currently provide full-text articles free-of-charge. If access is made from a subscribed library, journal articles can be downloaded. (Subscribers must first download the software named CNKI reader.) The database contains over 100 Chinese medical journals. For the full list, visit http://online.eastview .com/cnki_login/index.jsp (English, through East View Online Services). Through the Wanfang Database and the China National Knowledge Infrastructure, 90 percent of Chinese medical journals can be found.

Chinese Medical Association
http://www.cma.org.cn/artClass.asp?ClassID = 34
Chinese (simplified)

The Chinese Medical Association publishes a series of journals on Chinese medicine, introductions to which are published on this Web site. Readers can search the full-text articles and the tables of contents through the Wanfang Database.

Chinese Medicine, Chinese Herbal Medicine and Acupuncture Medline
http://www.famouschinese.com/jsp/medline/chinese_medicine_medline.html
English

This searchable database draws its contents directly from Medline/PubMed data (U.S. National Library of Medicine) and has filtered that information for researchers interested in Chinese medicine and herbs. There are quick links on the main page to lists of results on subjects like traditional oriental medicine, acupuncture, and moxibustion. Users can search by typing in keywords. The Web site also provides the most recent research articles from Medline for Chinese medicine, Chinese Herbal Medicine, and Acupuncture.

Chinese Medicine Journal Title Search
http://hint.nhri.org.tw/cgi-bin/flyweb/cmed.cgi?o = d3&u = 1_9100_Z1_flysheet
Chinese (traditional)

A search system is established by the National Chinese Medicine Research Institute. Users can search for articles in the *Chinese Medicine Journal* by typing in keywords.

Chinese Science Document Service System
http://sciencechina.cn/
Chinese (simplified)

Users can search for articles on Chinese journals for a fee.

ClinicalTrials.gov
http://clinicaltrials.gov/ct
English

Developed by the National Library of medicine, ClinicalTrials.gov provides regularly updated information about federally and privately supported clinical research in human volunteers. ClinicalTrials.gov gives you information about a trial's purpose, who may participate, locations, and phone numbers for more details. Clinical research on Chinese medicine and acupuncture can be found on the site. This free-of-charge database offers very detailed information.

Cochrane Collaboration
http://www.cochrane.org
English

The Cochrane Library is a service of the Cochrane Collaboration, an international nonprofit organization. This online library includes numerous databases about the effects of health care and is updated four times a year. The interested researcher can access the Cochrane Reviews from the library Web site free of charge. Abstracts and summaries are searchable by topic or by title, although for access to the entire article, the user needs to subscribe to the Cochrane Library or pay-per-view. Abstracts of the reviews can be viewed at no charge at the Collaboration's Web site (http://www.cochrane.org/cochrane/revabstr/mainindex.htm). The Cochrane Library includes information from databases such as the NHS Economic Evaluation Database and the Health Technology Assessment Database. Searches can be done by and results can be limited to "topic," "only new reviews," "only updated reviews," "full list by title," "NeLH 'Little Gems'," "Evidence Aid Summaries," "Cochrane Methodology abstracts," and "Abstracts in Spanish." Among the essays found in *Cochrane Reviews,* there are many studies regarding acupuncture. The complete text can be read on the Cochrane Library Web site with a fee. Users can browse and search abstracts of reviews free of charge. The author tried to search for "acupuncture," and 129 entries with plain language summary or abstract are resulted.

Database of Abstracts of Reviews of Effects
http://www.york.ac.uk/inst/crd/crddatabases.htm#DARE
English

Created in 1994 by the Center for Reviews and Dissemination at the University of York, the database covers a variety of health care topics and is particularly strong in resources on the effects of interventions. This is one of the databases that is included in the Cochrane Library. The reviews available in the database summarize and synthesize information available in peer-reviewed publications. Links to the original publications are often provided in the review or abstract.

Directory of Open Access Journals
http://www.doaj.org/
English

The Directory of Open Access Journals was created to assist researchers in locating and reading full-text articles that have been published in edited or peer-reviewed journals that do not require payment for access. This database is searchable by journal title, subject, and keywords. At the present time, over 2,800 journals comprising over 140,000 articles are indexed in this database with over 800 journals that can be searched.

The Web site, maintained by Lund University library, Sweden, has a search engine to find journals and articles by keyword, subject or title.

Dissertation and Thesis Abstract System
http://etds.ncl.edu.tw/theabs/index.jsp
Chinese (traditional) and English

The site is a database collecting all dissertations and theses from all universities in Taiwan. Theses written in English on Chinese medicine can be found through the service of UMI ProQuest (http://wwwlib.umi.com/dissertations). Health Science Library System of Pittsburgh University also creates a Web site named "Recent Dissertation in Medical Humanities." (http://www.hsls .pitt.edu/guides/histmed/researchresources/dissertations/index_ html).

Echo
http://echo.gmu.edu/center.php
English

Created in 2001 by the Center for History and New Media at George Mason University, the Echo Research Center has collected over 5,000 Web sites that cover a variety of topics such as science, medicine, and technology, and span all historical periods. Each site is reviewed and annotated, and then entered into the database. Included is a link to the original Web site, an extract that summarizes the key aspects of that Web site, and a list of keywords and annotations.

FindArticles
http://www.findarticles.com/
English

FindArticles gives you free access to millions of articles from thousands of top publications. The Web site is a database. Users can find and read relevant essays by searching with TCM keywords like "acupuncture" and "Chinese medicine."

Formosan Medical Association Journal Database
http://www.tbmc.com.tw/tbmc2/tbmce/B-11.htm
Chinese (traditional) and English

The Web site collects the complete text of articles published in the journals of the Formosan Medical Association between 1902 and 1945. A search function is available with a paid registration.

High Beam
http://www.highbeam.com/
English

High Beam is a (pay) search site that archives magazine, newspaper, and online news articles from the past twenty years. It boasts indexing of over 3,000 sources such as major U.S. newspapers, book reviews, and peer-reviewed journals.

International Bibliographic Information on Dietary
Supplements Database
http://ods.od.nih.gov/showpage.aspx?pageid = 48
English

The International Bibliographic Information on Dietary Supplements (IBIDS) database provides access to bibliographic citations and abstracts from published, international, and scientific literature on dietary supplements. The Office of Dietary Supplements at the National Institutes of Health produces this database to help consumers, health care providers, educators, and researchers find credible, scientific information on a variety of dietary supplements including vitamins, minerals, and botanicals. Users can choose to search the Full IBIDS Database, a subset of Consumer Citations Only or Peer Reviewed Citations Only. The Web site gives a detailed introduction on the database. Information on Chinese herbal medicine can be found.

Longyuan Journal Site
http://cn.qikan.com/
Chinese (simplified)

The Web site collects twenty-five Chinese medicine journals, like *Chinese Medicine and Pharmacology Journal, Chinese Acupuncture, Zhejiang Chinese Medicine and Pharmacology Journal.* It provides the tables of contents of the latest and past issues. Users can pay for articles in full text.

Manual Alternative and Natural Therapy Index System
http://www.chiroaccess.com/MANTISDatabaseOverview.html
http://www.fcer.org/html/Member/MantisJournals.htm
English

MANTIS is a database that indexes alternative medical literature, which provides citations and abstracts. It boasts information from over 1,000 journals from 1900 to the present day. The aim of MANTIS is to provide evidence-based information from peer-reviewed journals to practitioners of both Western and traditional medicine. Some of the focuses of MANTIS include acupuncture, herbal medicine, Moxibustion, massage, traditional oriental medicine, and homeopathy, although the main focus is on chiropractic. Approximately 70 percent of the references include abstracts. A subscription is needed to search MANTIS. The Web site publishes the journal list of the database. As seen from the list, the database has collected many journals related to Chinese medicine. The database is only available for a fee.

MedBio World
http://www.sciencekomm.at/
English

MedBio World was founded in the mid 1990s in Australia. It is a Web site that provides resources on medical and biological sciences. The four tools offered by this Web site are Health News Explorer, MedBio News, MedBio Access, and a Genomics Blog. The Health News Explorer feature collects and indexes over 40,000 articles from Reuter's Health. Simple search capabilities allow the user to query for articles on a variety of topics. The results page offers article title, date, and a brief summary. This service is free to users. The Web site provides free searches for articles, books and abstracts by typing in keywords. Users will have to pay for full-text articles.

MedlinePlus
http://www.nlm.nih.gov/medlineplus/medlineplus.html
English

MedlinePlus will direct you to information to help answer health questions. MedlinePlus brings together authoritative information from NLM, the National Institutes of Health, and other government agencies and health-related organizations. Preformulated Medline searches are included in MedlinePlus and give easy access to medical journal articles. MedlinePlus also has extensive information about drugs, an illustrated medical encyclopedia, interactive patient tutorials, and the latest health news.

National Research Institute of Chinese Medicine
http://nricm1.nricm.edu.tw/textdb.php
Chinese (traditional)

The National Research Institute of Chinese Medicine offers access to a variety of databases, such as the Institute of Chinese Medicine Database. These databases include information from Chinese medical journals, as well as magazines and journals on Chinese medicine. Registered users can gain access to sites on medical journals of Mainland China. Many of the databases are accessible after registration, with the exception of medical journals from Mainland China, which can only be accessed at the Institute.

National Science and Technology Library
http://www.nstl.gov.cn/index.html
Chinese (simplified)

Established in 2000, National Science and Technology Library is a virtual information center that provides Chinese and English full-text conference articles and a dissertations delivery service for free. The site contains journals and dissertations of Chinese and English retrieval system.

PerioPath: Index to Chinese Periodical Literature
http://readopac2.ncl.edu.tw/ncl3/index.jsp
Chinese (traditional) and English

PerioPath is an online index created and maintained by the National Central Library of the Republic of China. It contains information on articles from approximately 2,600 Chinese and Western language periodicals published in Taiwan, Hong Kong, and Macau from 1994. Users can search for articles under title, author, class code, keyword, journal title, or publication date. The database contains twenty-five Chinese medical journals published in Taiwan.

PubMed (National Library of Medicine)
http://www.ncbi.nlm.nih.gov/PubMed
English

PubMed is a service of the U.S. National Library of Medicine that includes over 16 million citations from Medline and other life science journals for biomedical articles back to the 1950s. PubMed includes links to full-text articles and other related resources. PubMed provides online access to journals on Chinese medicine such as *Chinese Medical Journal, Chinese Journal of Traumatology,* and *The American Journal of Chinese Medicine.* Users can simply enter keywords to search for relevant studies on Chinese medicine published in these journals. PubMed also provides an index of Chinese medicine journals in Chinese, which can be searched by entering the appropriate Pinyin.

The Complete Collection of Online Journals
http://zazhi.zcom.com/
Chinese (simplified)

The Web site introduces Chinese journals. Under the "Chinese Medicine" category, it lists forty titles of TCM journals and their brief introductions without tables of contents, abstracts or full text.

WanFang Database
http://www.wanfangdata.com.cn (Chinese)
http://www.periodicals.net.cn/english.html (English)
Chinese (simplified and traditional) and English

The database contains ninety Chinese medical journals, which are listed at http://www.periodicals.net.cn/eqikan.asp?codeID = R. The section "Medicines and Hygiene" contains most journals about Chinese medicine published in China. Except for the series of medical journals published by the Chinese Medical Association, the site contains journals published by most universities of Chinese medicine. Full-text journals can be accessed by subscribers. Tables of contents are available to the public.

Through the Wanfang Database and the China National Knowledge Infrastructure, 90 percent of Chinese medical journals can be found.

Wei Pu Information
http://newweb.cqvip.com
Chinese (simplified)

The Web site is the "Chinese Science and Technology Journal Database," which collects Chinese science and technology journals published in Mainland China. It includes 162 categories of Chinese medicine journals, which can be searched by two separated periods of 2000-2006 and 1989-1999. Users can search by keywords, author, title or journal name, and basic information will be shown. To read the complete text, users must pay for registration.

Other Search Engines

The following are Web sites search for medicine- related articles, books, and reports. Users can search by keywords. Most results come with free abstracts. Users will have to pay for full-text articles, except for some journals that give free access.

Chinese Biological Abstracts
http://www.cba.ac.cn/
Chinese (simplified)

The database collects more than 800 journals, covering biological sciences, medicine, and pharmacology. The collection started at 1985. This database also includes reviews, reports, and dissertations. The Web site is only an introduction to the CD-Rom version and online version of the database.

Ebsco-Academic Search Premier
http://search.epnet.com
English

IngentaConnect: The Home of Scholarly Research
http://www.ingentaconnect.com/
English

Online Computer Library Center
http://www.oclc.org
English

Enabled by FirstSearch, users can find and retrieve materials on almost any research topic. The service delivers bibliographic records and library holdings from WorldCat, electronic journals from Electronic Collections Online, and access to more than seventy-two databases to give users a convenient and easy-to-use reference service that is searchable in five languages. The center was founded in 1967 as a service for libraries and researchers. They created and currently maintain WorldCat, an international library catalog, and Electronic Collections Online, which provides access to 9,000 full-text journals, and more than 4,000 full-image journals in numerous languages online. Many college and university libraries around the world subscribe to the centers features and provide access to WorldCat to their students, staff, and faculty.

Ovid: a Wolters Kluwer Business
http://www.ovid.com/site/index.jsp
English

SpringerLink
http://springerlink.metapress.com/home/main.mpx
English

ProQuest Medical Library
http://www.proquest.com/products_pq/descriptions/pq_
  medical_library.shtml
English

Sage Journal Online
http://online.sagepub.com
English

ScienceDirect
http://www.sciencedirect.com/
English

Wiley Interscience
http://www.interscience.wiley.com
English

BIBLIOGRAPHIES

Bibliography of Western Publications on the History of Chinese Science and Medicine
http://ccat.sas.upenn.edu/~nsivin/nakbib.html
English

> This bibliography was written by Dr. Nathan Sivin, professor emeritus of Chinese culture and the history of science, at the University of Pennsylvania. Dr. Sivin's list emphasizes recent publications. With respect to China, before about 1800, the bibliographies that can be found in Joseph Needham's Science and Civilisation in China are extremely rich and merely need to be supplemented. Although Sivin's references are largely unannotated, the reader can easily use the indexes to find evaluations of sources. There is no corresponding thorough survey for the last two centuries, but a large part of the literature on that period published more than a decade ago is already obsolete. Books on traditional medicine are published, most of them with no scholarly value, because medicine is still widely practiced and because the commercial demand both within and outside of China is enormous. Historians have conspicuously neglected recent technology and science. Most publications on this list deal with policy rather than the work itself and the researchers. Publications are included mostly because of their quality and usefulness, a few are included in order to warn readers that the promise of their titles is specious. The bibliography covers the following topics, each closely related to TCM: "Alchemy and Early Chemical Arts," "History of Medicine in Imperial China," "Medicine and Related Topics," "*Materia Medica*," "History of Medicine in Twentieth-century China."

Bibliography of Western-Language Sources on Acupuncture
http://www.akupunkturdoktor.dk/dokumentation/index.asp
Danish and English

The bibliography is listed according to the following topics: "Methods of Acupuncture," "Trigger point acupuncture," "A new system of acupuncture," "Mechanisms of acupuncture," "Acupuncture's non-segmental and segmental analgesic effects: The point of meridians," "Segmental acupuncture," "Acupuncture and the peripheral nervous system," "Electroacupuncture and acupuncture analgesia," "Transcutaneous electrical nerve stimulation," "Laser therapy," "The clinical evaluation of the acupuncture," "The clinical use of, and evidence for, acupuncture in the medical systems," "Acupuncture for nausea and vomiting," "Acupuncture in the pain clinic," "Acupuncture for rheumatological problems," "Acupuncture for the withdrawal of habituating substances," "Adverse reactions to acupuncture," and "Reinterpretation of traditional concepts in acupuncture."

Bibliography of Western-Language Sources on Medicine in East Asia
http://www.albion.edu/history/chimed/eambiblio/eambib.html
English

Compiled by Marta Hanson, with contributions from Yi-Li Wu, the bibliography lists titles according to the following topics: "Asian Medicine: General," "Chinese Medicine: History and Anthropology," "Western Medicine in China," "Translations of Chinese Medical Texts," "Chinese Materia Medica and Botany," "Traditional Chinese Medicine: popular introductions to practice," "Traditional Chinese Medicine: clinical textbooks for practitioners," "T'ai Chi Ch'uan translated texts and practice," "Journals and Newsletters of Interest," "Medicine in Japan: History and Anthropology," and "Medicine in Korea: Anthropology."

CORK Bibliography: Acupuncture
http://www.projectcork.org/bibliographies/data/Bibliography_
Acupuncture.html
English

The Web site provides fifty-two citations from articles regarding acupuncture, published since 1997, each attached with an abstract.

Current Bibliographies in Medicine: Acupuncture
http://www.nlm.nih.gov/archive/20040823/pubs/cbm/
acupuncture.html
English

This site includes a total of 2,302 citations, from January 1970 through October 1997. It is prepared by Lori J. Klein, MALS, National Library of Medicine and Alan I. Trachtenberg, MD, MPH, National Institute on Drug Abuse. The Web site was first established in October 1997. Users can search its contents according to the following topics: "Addictions and Psychiatric Disorders," "Allergy and Immunology," "Auricular (Ear) Acupuncture," "Biochemistry and Physiology," "Cardiovascular System," "Dermatology," "Face, Sinuses, Mouth, and Throat," "Gastroenterology," "General Pain," "Genitourinary, Pelvic, and Reproductive Systems," "Headache," "Low Back, Sciatica," "Lower Extremities," "Miscellaneous," "Nausea, Vomiting, and Postoperative Problems," "Neck and Shoulders," "Nervous System and Special Senses," "Research Methods," "Reviews," "Side Effects," "Upper Extremities and Breast," "Veterinary Medicine," "Who, What, When, Where" and "Additional Books in English."

Solving Scientific and Medical Problems in General Research on China
http://ccat.sas.upenn.edu/~nsivin/scimed.html
English

> Compiled by Dr. Nathan Sivin, the bibliography covers the following topics, each closely related to TCM: "The Human Body," "Health and Illness," "Plants," "Animals," "Minerals," "Elixirs and other Accoutrements of Immortality." The last update was in November, 2005.

Western-language Studies on Chinese Alchemy
http://venus.unive.it/dsao/pregadio/tools/biblio/biblio_0.html
English

> This is an updated version of a bibliography first published in Monumenta Serica 44 (1996): 439-476. An earlier, not updated version (with entries arranged in alphabetical order) is available as a single file via FTP (ftp://coombs.anu.edu.au/coombspapers/subj-bibl-clearinghouse/chinese-alchemy-bibl.txt) from the Coombspapers Archive, Australian National University.
>
> The contents are divided into several categories: "Introduction," "General Studies," "Studies of Alchemical Texts and Authors," "Studies of Specific Features."

Electronic Texts

Bencao Gang Mu
http://www.haokucn.com/search/data/Html_data/bcgm/index.htm
Chinese (simplified)

> Li Shizhen's *Bencao Gang Mu* is the most comprehensive medical book; it includes 1,892 substances, 10,000 prescriptions, collecting methods, herb processing, and combined use in formulae for each medicine. It is difficult for users to search the

contents because the book has fifty-two volumes. This site is a
database of Bencao Gang Mu and the full text can be read and
searched. There are many color pictures of substances on this
Web site.

Chinese Ancient Texts Database
http://www.chant.org/
Chinese (traditional)

Developed by the Research Center for Chinese Ancient Texts
of the Chinese University of Hong Kong, the software aims to
build up an electronic database of all traditional and excavated
Chinese ancient texts. Currently all ancient texts prior to the
Six Dynasties (AD 589) are included in the database. Users can
pay for registration and search the database online. A free trial
version is available.

Chinese Medical Classics
http://www.tcmbook.cn/
Chinese (simplified and traditional)

The Web site provides more than 700 Chinese Medical Classics. The contents can be searched with a fee. Chinese Medical
Classics also has a CD version.

Chinese Medical Literature
http://bencao.cintcm.ac.cn/index.htm
Chinese (simplified)

Maintained by Chinese Medical Sciences Data Center, the Web
site collates ancient medical literature and digitizes them. The
site has discussions on the digitization of ancient medical literature. The site also offers a free database, titled Ancient Chinese
Medical Literature Knowledge Database, which includes twelve
kinds of ancient medical literature (such as *Materia Medica,*
acupuncture, diagnosis, nourishing life, formulae, shang han,
case studies, and medical history).

Chinese Medical Treasure Garden
http://jvzhuo.51.net/index.htm
http://juzhuo.go1.icpcn.com
Chinese (simplified)

The Web site claims to provide hundreds of Chinese medical classics in complete texts. However, when the author browsed the Web site, none of the text is downloadable. Some of the texts are readable online.

Chinese Medicine Classical Treatise
http://www.chinapage.com/medicine/medicine.html
English

The complete online text of *Su wen, Ling shu, Nan jing, Shennong bencao jing, Jin gui yao lue, Ge Hong's Bao Po Zi Nei Pian* (The inner chapter of Bao Po Zi), *Zhang Zhongjing's Shang han lun* and *Bian Que's Cang Gong Lie Zhuan* (Biography of Bianque).

Chinese Medicine Clinical Base
http://zylc.njutcm.edu.cn/xuekedatabase.asp
Chinese (simplified)

Maintained by Nanjing University of TCM, the site offers thirteen Chinese medical classics, including medical classics, Chinese *Materia Medica* and case studies, for viewing online. It also contains databases of "Wen bing" literature, terms of Wen bing, terms of Shang han lun, and terms of Jin gui yao lue, respectively. These databases can be searched online for free.

Ancient Chinese Medical Classics
http://www.ccmp.gov.tw/public/public.asp?selno = 525&relno = 525
Chinese (traditional)

The Web site provides over eighty ancient Chinese medical classics for free download such as *Huangdi neijing, Ju fang fa hui*

(Elucidation of Formularies of the Bureau), *Zhen jiu da cheng* (Great Compendium of Acupuncture and Moxibustion), *Bencao Gang Mu,* and *Yi zong jin jian* (Golden Mirror of Medicine).

Electronic Classical Texts in Chinese Medicine
http://www.tcmet.com.tw
Chinese (traditional)

This site is a database about traditional Chinese medical texts including *Huangdi neijing, Collection of Li Gao, Collection of Lui Hejian, Collection of Zhang Congzheng, Collection of Zhu Zhenheng* and *Collection of Zhang Jiebin.* Furthermore, the full texts of *Huangdi neijing, Jin yuan si da jia* (The Four Great Masters of Jin and Yuan periods), *Jing yue quan shu* (Jing Yue's Complete Compendium) *Zhong yi yao ming ci hui bian* (Terminology in Chinese medicine), *Zhong yi shi yi wen xian hui bian* (Collection of Documents on Chinese Medicine and Epidemics), and *Zhongguo li dai chuan ran bing jiang yi* (Notes on Epidemic Diseases in Chinese History) can be searched and downloaded. Recently, prescriptions from *Bei Ji Qian Jin Fang* (Prescriptions Worth a Thousand Gold for Emergency) and *Collection of Lui Hejian* have been selected and placed on the Web site. Moreover, detailed explanations of *Huangdi neijing* and works by the Four Great Masters and *Zhang Jingyue* are given in the "Study Guide for Ancient Chinese Medical Literature."

Japanese Pharmacopoeia
http://jpdb.nihs.go.jp/jp14e/
English

This is the English version of the *Japanese Pharmacopoeia,* fourteenth edition. The Web site offers the complete text of the book in downloadable PDF format for free.

Full-text Database for Electronic Ancient Chinese Medical Texts, Capital Medical University Library
http://read.freeduan.com/data/2006/0530/article_2647.htm
Chinese (simplified)

The site provides thirty-four Chinese medical texts, written during Ming and Qing periods, for free. Readers have to download CAJ Reader in order to read the texts.

Gu Jin Tu Shu Ji Cheng and Si Ku Quan Shu
http://www.greatman.com.tw/database.htm
Chinese (traditional)

Gu jin tu shu ji cheng (The Complete Collection of Ancient and Modern Books) and *Si ku quan shu* (The Compendium of the Four Vaults) are the biggest collection of books in Chinese history. *Si ku quan shu* is divided into four parts: Classics, Histories, Masters, and Collections. Medical classics are collected in the Masters.

Gu jin tu shu ji cheng has a section on medicine. The two collections have gathered all ancient medical classics in Chinese history. This database has included these two collections for data search. Users have to purchase the database, but free trials are available online.

Guo Xue Bao Dian
http://www.gxbd.com/index.html?op = 6&id = 3e
Chinese (simplified)

The site provides the full-texts of fifteen medical classics such as *Su wen, Nan jing, Ling hsu, Jin gui yao lue, Shennong bencao jing*, etc. The Web site indicates the versions of each specific text used. Users can search through the contents after paying a fee.

Harikyu.com
http://www.harikyu.com/general/data/edu.html
http://www.harikyu.com/general/data/ko-otu.txt
http://www.harikyu.com/general/data/11.txt
http://www.harikyu.com/general/data/myaku2.txt
Japanese

This Web site provides free electronic versions of *Zhen jiu jia yi jing* (The Classic ABCs of Acupuncture and Moxibustion), Zu bi shi yi mai jiu jing (Cauterization of the Eleven Vessels of the Foot and Forearm), *Yin yang shi yi mai jiu jing* (Cauterization Canon of the Eleven Yin and Yang Vessels), *Zhang jia shan han jian mai shu* and(Western Han Bamboo Strip "book on the pulse" from Zhangjiashan). The Web site has links to other medical classics, (but these links lead to pages not found). *Zu bi shi yi mai jiu jing* and *Yin yang shi yi mai jiu jing* were unearthed from a Mawangdui grave from the second century BC in Hunan Province in 1973. Their contents include medical theories, drugs, and physical exercise.

Scripta Sinica
http://www.sinica.edu.tw/~tdbproj/handy1/
Chinese (traditional)

This database of complete ancient Chinese texts set up by the Academia Sinica of Taiwan includes Twenty-five Histories, Thirteen Canons, Taoist canons, Buddhist sutras, and thirty-one other ancient classics. All literature can be searched online for free.

Sheng Wu Gu
http://www.bioon.com/Article/Class193/Index.shtml
Chinese (simplified)

The site offers many important Chinese medical classics online such as *Shennong bencao jing, Huangdi neijing, Jing yue quan shu, Shang han lun, Wai ke zheng zong, Yi lin gai cuo* (correcting mistakes in TCM), just to name a few.

Selected Edition of the Compendium of Materia Medica
http://www.duosuccess.com/BZGM/001a04080101.htm
Chinese (traditional)

The site provides part of the *Bencao gang mu* online.

The Chinese Medical Classics World
http://211.23.187.10/medicine/main.asp
Chinese (traditional)

The Web site provides selections from more than seventy Chinese medical classics and a formulae search.

Zhu bing yuan hou lun
http://aeam.umin.ac.jp/siryouko/syobyogenkoron.htm
Japanese and Chinese (traditional)

The complete online text of *Zhu bing yuan hou lun* (Origin and Indicators of Disease) complied in Sui dynasty (AD 581-618).

NOTES

1. Zhan, Youxiang et al., Development and utilization of medical information resource in China. <www.ifla.org/IV/ifla70/papers/017e-Youxiang_Jiving.pdf> ; Ji, Z.L. et al. (2006). Traditional Chinese Medicine information database, *Journal of Ethnopharmacology 103*(3): 501. Pak Kwan Hui et al. (2003). Information system in Chinese medicine. In PC Leung et al (eds.), *A Comprehensive Guide to Chinese Medicine,* Singapore: World Scientific Press, pp. 325-342.
2. See <www.cintcm.com> and <www.cintcm.ac.cn> .
3. Yi Feng et al. (2006). Knowledge discovery in Traditional Chinese Medicine: State of the art and perspectives, *Artificial Intelligence in Medicine, 38*(3): 219-236.
4. TCM Online Web site <www.cintcm.com/> .

5. Hoffecker, Lilian et al. (2006). A review of seven complementary and alternative medicine databases. *Journal of Electronic Resources in Medical Libraries 3*(4): 13-31.

6. Lee, Simon Ming and Yuen, et al. (2003). Biochemistry and herbs. In P.C. Leung et al., *A Comprehensive Guide to Chinese Medicine*, pp. 113-142. For interesting example, see Buenz, Eric J. et al. (2006). Searching historical herbal texts for potential new drugs. *British Medical Journal 333:* 1314-1315. <www.bmj.com/cgi/content/full/333/7582/1314>. Bakalar, Nicholas (2007). 17th-Century remedy; 21st-Century potency, *New York Times,* January 16 2007. <www.nytimes.com/2007/01/16/health/16herb .html?_r = 1&ex = 157680000&en = aef393d877c555c5&ei = 5124& partner = permalink&exprod = permalink&oref = slogin> .

Chapter 7

History and Philosophy

Traditional Chinese Medicine has undergone a long course of development and witnessed the emergence of a great number of highly skilled and talented doctors who made brilliant medical achievements. Learning about the course of Chinese medical history is an invaluable experience for students who are learning Chinese medicine. In many TCM programs in schools around the world, the history of Chinese medicine is a fundamental and often compulsory course. Readers may wonder about the significance of Chinese medical history. Chinese medicine, which continues to develop from ancient times to the present, documents and records in an ancient writing tradition that is at the same time evolving as medical concepts are evolving. Learning medical classics is a significant step in understanding and knowing medical theories and clinical cases. For example, although *Huangdi neijing, Shennong bencao jing,* and *Shang han lun* were written over 1,000 years ago, the theories recorded in these classics are still practiced by modern physicians. Therefore, learning medical classics, to some extent, is the best way to learn Chinese medicine. Chinese medical history is like a key for the door to the myriad treasures of Chinese medicine.

Asian Society for the History of Medicine
http://www.ihp.sinica.edu.tw/~medicine/ashm/
Chinese (traditional) and English

This is a membership organization open to anyone interested in the history of Oriental medicine anywhere in the world. The society was founded in 2001 as a way for medical historians around the world to meet and share information in a collegial environment. Topics of interest to the society include historical perspectives into public health, pharmacy, dentistry, nursing, and medicine in Asian countries. Meetings are organized biannually, and a newsletter is released semiannually. The society also keeps a database of medical historians active in this research field. The society plans to organize meetings once every two years, to issue a newsletter every six months, and maintain a registry of medical historians in Asia. The site provides news, forums, links to history of medicine sites, and a directory of scholars. The site has information about conferences held by the Asian Society for the History of Medicine.

Bencao, Yaoxue and Bowu: the formation of Traditional Chinese Medicine
http://saturn.ihp.sinica.edu.tw/~bencao/
Chinese (traditional)

This site was created for the research project titled "Bencao, Yaoxue and Bowu"(the Formation of Traditional Chinese Medicine) conducted by the Research Group of the History of Health and Healing, Institute of History and Philology, Academia Sinica, Taiwan. Professor Jianmin Li is the chief researcher of this project and the manager of the site. The aim of the project is to explain and discuss three important classical texts, *Shang han lun, Zheng lei bencao* (Classified *Materia Medica* compiled in Song dynasty), and *Bencao gang mu,* under the cooperation of historians, sociologists, and other scholars of Chinese medical literature, to explore the formation, development and transmission of crucial medical concepts. It posts a variety of academic announcements, activities, news, research, courses in the history of *Materia Medica,* and databases. Interested scholars will find this database useful since references and journals can be found. Furthermore, Dr. Li regularly invites scholars in this field to present their latest research.

Center for Science and Technology Resources, National Tsing-hua University
http://www.lib.nthu.edu.tw/STS/index.html
Chinese (traditional)

One of the reasons for National Tsing-hua University to establish its Center for Science and Technology Resources was to collect sources on the history of science. The site introduces the collections and databases of the center, and it provides bibliographies for books on history of science and technology written in Chinese, English, and Japanese languages, respectively.

ChiMed: The History of Chinese Medicine Webpage
http://www.albion.edu/history/chimed/
English

ChiMed is an online resource for researchers interested in the history of Chinese medicine. The site includes both a directory of scholars working in the field of the history of Chinese medicine, as well as universities around the world that teach the subject. Links to international libraries that have a large number of titles on the history of Chinese medicine are provided, as well as links to online journals and electronic resources. A few bibliographies and course syllabi have also been shared on the site. It provides a variety of resources, categorized by subjects, including directory of scholars, institutions, libraries, online and electronic resources, bibliographies and syllabi, news, and events. The directory of scholars lists the specialties and contact information (addresses, and e-mails) of scholars all over the world. The news and events section offers information about scholarships, conferences, seminars, forthcoming publications, and so on. All in all, anyone who is interested in the history of Chinese medicine cannot afford to ignore this Web site. It is one of the major online resources of Chinese Medicine for historians. This site is hosted at Albion College in Michigan.

Chinese Medical Classics Text Series
http://venus.unive.it/pregadio/ikei.html
http://helios.unive.it/~pregadio/ikei.html
http://www.chinesemedicinedoc.com/index.php?page = classic_
  texts
http://aeam.umin.ac.jp/siryouko/index.htm
Chinese (traditional) and English

The site, maintained by Fabrizio Pregadio, offers electronic versions of Chinese medical classics, including *Su wen, Ling shu, Nan jing, Shang han lun, Jin gui yao lue. Shennong bencao jing,* and *Bian que cang gong lie zhuan* (Biography of Bianque). The page also states the formats and the editions of each text. This Web site has uploaded seven medical classics online. Users may search content by the browser's search function.

Chinese Medicinals
http://www.hort.purdue.edu/newcrop/proceedings1990/v1-499
  .html
English

This site is maintained by Albert Leung. It mainly introduces the history of Chinese medicine with references to related classical texts. In the Web site, Leung lists many related books and journals published in Mainland China. The site covers history, contemporary sources of information on Chinese medicine, scope of Chinese *Materia Medica,* and examples of common Chinese medicinals. A good guide for those who want to learn about both ancient and modern Chinese medicinals.

Chinese Medicine History
http://www.taijichinesemedicine.com/TCMhistory.htm
English

This is a rather introductory site. The site lists twenty-eight famous physicians in Chinese history with very brief biographies attached with graphic images.

The content of the Web site is brief, which is suitable for TCM history beginners.

Chinese Public Health Posters
http://clendening.kumc.edu/dc/cp/
English

This site offers twenty-five posters about Chinese public health in republican China with English translation.

Chinese Society for the History of Science and Technology
http://www.ihns.ac.cn/xuehui/society.htm
Chinese (Simplified)

The site provides information of the society, including an introduction to the society, its academic activities, its newsletter, and its achievements. The Web site provides rich information on the history of Chinese technology.

Classics of Traditional Chinese Medicine- NLM, History of Medicine Div.
http://www.nlm.nih.gov/hmd/chinese/chinesehome.html
English

The National Library of Medicine (NLM) holds approximately 2,000 volumes of Chinese medical classics. Here we display a few of the earliest and most interesting texts from the NLM collection. Also included are portraits of a few significant figures in early Chinese medicine whose contributions range from acupuncture to the pioneering uses of herbal medicines to the concept of Yin and Yang. Only one page of each of the thirteen medical books from China, Japan, and Korea are scanned.

Emotional Counter-Therapy
http://ccat.sas.upenn.edu/~nsivin/counter.pdf
English

The paper, a research article written by Dr. Nathan Sivin, introduces emotional counter-therapy in Chinese medical history.

Harikyu.com
http://www.harikyu.com/general/data/edu.html
Japanese

This Web site provides free electronic versions of *Zhen jiu jia yi jing* (The classic ABCs of acupuncture and moxibustion), *Zu bi shi yi mai jiu jing* (Cauterization of the Eleven Vessels of the Foot and Forearm), *Yin yang shi yi mai jiu jing* (Cauterization Canon of the Eleven Yin and Yang Vessels), *Zhang jia shan han jian mai shu* (Western Han Bamboo Strip "book on the pulse" from Zhangjiashan). It links to other medical classics, (but these links lead to pages not found). *Zu bi shi yi mai jiu jing* and *Yin yang shi yi mai jiu jing* were unearthed from a Mawangdui grave from the second century BC in Hunan Province in 1973. Their contents include medical theories, drugs, and physical exercise.

History of Images and Medicine
http://www.ihp.sinica.edu.tw/~medicine/ih/
Chinese (traditional)

This is the Web site of the project "History of Images and Medicine."

The project studies pictures and images related to the history of medicine, with an emphasis placed on graphs and images of human bodies, acupoints, medicine, and Daoist magical charms. The Web site provides news on the research project, and in its "Image database," users can find images of internal organs in medical books.

History of Traditional Chinese Medicine
http://medhist.kams.or.kr/index_e.html
English

Established by the Karolinska Institute, this site provides links
to other sites that are about the history of Traditional Chinese
Medicine. However, many provided links are rather irrelevant to
the history of Chinese medicine. There is no category organizing the provided links, making the Web site less user friendly.
Also, it is not frequently updated.

International Society for the History of East Asian Science
   Technology and Medicine
http://www.nri.org.uk/ISHEASTM.html
English

The society was founded in 1990 with the dual goal of serving
and representing researchers interested in the history of Eastern Asia, in particular, science, technology, and medicine. The
society holds a triennial conference at various international locations, and it produces a journal called *East Asian Science,
Technology, and Medicine*. In addition, the newsletter of the
society can be found on the site.

Japan Society of Acupuncture and Moxibustion History
http://homepage3.nifty.com/rinbunkai/
Japanese

The Japan Society of Acupuncture and Moxibustion History is
an academic association specializing in acupuncture. Its Web
site provides news, publications, and seminar notices of the
Society.

Japan Society of Medical History (JSMH)
http://flcsvr.rc.kyushu-u.ac.jp/~michel/jsmh/
Japanese and English

The Japan Society of Medical History was organized in 1892 under the guidance of Yu Fujikawa, a famous scholar in the field of Japanese medical history. The society is the most important organization in the field of the history of medicine in Japan. The Japan Society of Medical History holds a conference annually, and one of the important research topics is always the history of Chinese medicine. The Web site contains a history of the society, information on monthly meeting and events, a journal published by the JSMH, articles of association, annual congress, and a bibliography of the history of medicine in Japan in a variety of Western languages. This society studies Japanese and Chinese medicine, and it is known that Japanese medicine has been significantly influenced by, and is closely related to, Chinese medicine.

Japan Society for study of Neijing
http://plaza.umin.ac.jp/~daikei
Japanese

Huangdi neijing is the earliest medical classic in China and thus the fundamental classic of Chinese medicine. This society is an academic organization that specializes in *Huangdi neijing*. The Web site introduces the organization, its members, and news.

Marta Hanson's History of Medicine and Culture in China
http://japan.ucsd.edu/Marta/home/index.htm
English

Marta Hanson at the University of Maryland seeks to bring together information on research, teaching, academics, publication, and funding for scholars interested in the history of medicine in China. The teaching section includes lectures, seminars, syllabi, bibliographies, and databases, and the academic section features a list of conferences, societies, and associations. Dr. Hanson's section on research and publications is very thorough, with links to institutions, individuals, and publishers who deal with the history and practice of Chinese medicine. This is a comprehensive site. Dr. Marta Hanson lists her personal information, research, teaching courses, resources, and links for the history of science, technology, and medicine in East Asia on this Web site. This site collects useful links of syllabi, in which users can find bibliographies and references of Chinese medical history.

Materia medica sinica
http://www.materia-medica-sinica.de/
English

The site, entitled *"Materia medica sinica* Ethnophilological Studies in the Early History of the benaco-literature," publishes a paper titled *Philosophy and medicine: reflections of the Huai-nan tzu in the Compendium of Materia Medica of T'ao Hung-ching.* In this paper, the authors present a study on the relations between *Huai-nan tzu* and the *Compendium of materia medica.* The authors argued that, from Liang to Song, the quotations contained in the *Compendium of Materia Medica* were consciously drawn from *Huai-nan tzu,* in which the latter was cited as the *locus classicus.* However, hidden beneath these openly cited connections between pharmacology and philosophy lies a sea of pharmacological information that is both transmitted in *Huai-nan tzu* and in the earliest layers of the *Compendium of Materia Medica,* compiled by T'ao Hung-ching (456? to 536?). Surprisingly, parts of the pharmaco-philosophical interface between *Huai-nan tzu* and the *Compendium of Materia Medica* are transmitted as congruences. This is a very intensive article. This essay presented a very specialized study that would definitely advance the understanding of the history of Chinese Medicine. Nevertheless, the essay is targeted at those who have a solid understanding of TCM history.

Mayanagi's Laboratory for the History of Chinese Science
http://www.hum.ibaraki.ac.jp/chubun/mayanagi.html
Chinese and Japanese

Dr. Makoto Mayanagi is a professor of the College of Humanities, National Ibaraki University in Japan. His specialty is medical and pharmacological history in China and Japan. The site offers his course syllabus, databases, and links to other Web sites on the history of science in Japan. In addition, a searchable collection of his publications on the history of Chinese and Japanese medicine can be read online. This collection is the most important feature of the site. The site offers full-texts of Mayanagi's articles, which are professionally and knowledgeably written. These are very good articles for those who want to know more about history of Chinese medicine. The Japanese version is more detailed than the Chinese version

Medhist-China section
http://www.intute.ac.uk/healthandlifesciences/cgi-bin/browse_medhist.pl?id = 93897
English

Developed and managed by the Wellcome Library for the History and Understanding of Medicine at the Wellcome Trust, MedHist provides Web resources on a variety of topics in the history of medicine, health, and human development. This Web resource can be browsed under different topics, such as geographic location, disease, historical period, and electronic publications. MedHist is provided free of charge and publishes links to Web sites in addition to publishing evaluations of these sites. New entries are added regularly; the site would be of use to students, researchers, or anyone interested in the history of medicine. The Web site is categorized into "subjects," "personal names," "keywords," etc., making itself very user-friendly. Its columns, "what's new" and "event," report the latest news in the field of history of medicine. Nine Web sites are listed in the "China" section, and it is updated frequently. It has specialized editors to collect Web sites that satisfy the set criteria, and it guarantees the selected sites are of high quality and are written according to a standardized format.

Medicine, Healing and Body
http://sts.nthu.edu.tw/twmed
Chinese (traditional)

The Web site systematically categorizes resources about medicine, the history of medicine, and the history of the body on the Internet.

Museum of Digital Sources for Medical History of Taiwan
http://203.65.117.106/project/index.htm
Chinese (traditional)

The Web site introduces the medical history of Taiwan. It is divided into "Guide to Medicine in Taiwan," "Folk Healing Therapy," "Medical history of Customs and the Church," "Biographies of Significant Physicians," "Developmental History of Public Hygiene and Epidemic Prevention," "Nursing History," "Traditional Medicine," "Dental History," "History of Pharmacy." The comprehensive content of the Web site makes it an important source in understanding the medical history of Taiwan.

Needham Research Institute (NRI)
http://www.nri.org.uk/
English

The Needham Research Institute is located in Cambridge, England, and is a world-renowned center for the study of the science, medicine, and technology of East Asia. The library began in 1937 with collections from Joseph Needham, who became interested in this area of the world following WWII. He set up the NRI for promoting the study of Chinese science under his great project of Science and Civilization in China. Some of the rare books brought by Joseph Needham from the East deal with topics such as the history of Chinese medicine, archaeology, mathematics, and astronomy. Although the library's largest collection is from China, there are resources from Korea and Japan as well. There is online access to the library's catalog through subscription, however, there is an online version of Joseph Needham's archives available on the site as well. Other resources on the page include a newsletter and a link to interesting seminars and workshops. The NRI is a very important institute for promoting research into the history of Chinese medicine. There are five sections on the NRI page: first, an introduction to the life and contributions of Joseph Needham; second, the past, present, and future of the institute; third, the details of the project; fourth, an electronic version of the institute's newsletter; and fifth, a link to the East Asian History of Science Library home page, which was set up by Joseph Needham and which collects resources on East Asian science history. The site describes resources available at the institute. The library holds a great number of books, articles, and offprints. Through the Web page, users can search the library's catalog.

NRI is a major group involved in the history of Chinese medicine. In 2000, Nathan Sivin collected Needham's articles on the history of Chinese medicine into a book. In the same year, Hsing-tsung Huang joined the project and also published *Fermentations and Food Science* under the project in which "food and nutritional deficiency diseases" were discussed.

Religion and Healing
http://www.ihp.sinica.edu.tw/~linfs/rh/
Chinese (traditional)

This site is funded by Ministry of Education, Taiwan. The purpose of this project is to study the relationship between religions and healing in imperial China and Taiwan. The site provides news, research reports, and biographies of ancient Chinese doctors in pre-Han periods.

Religions, Medicine and Diet
http://www.sinica.edu.tw/~religion/
Chinese (traditional)

This is the Web site of the research project titled "Religions, Medicine and Diet." This research project focuses its attention on porridge in appreciation of its relationship with religion, medicine, and diet. Visitors can find news about the project. Most importantly, the Web site lists bibliographies on books regarding religions and medicine, and it has a good collection on sources on Buddhism and medicine.

Research group of the History of Health and Healing
http://www.ihp.sinica.edu.tw/%7Emedicine/
Chinese (traditional)

The Research Group of the History of Health and Healing is one of the research groups of the Institute of History and Philology at the Academia Sinica. This group focuses on the history of medicine and healing together with conceptions of health, sickness, and the body in China. The site contains monthly notices, events, conference news, classical texts, research notes, discussions, and a list of scholars. A research reference database of *Huangdi neijing* and the history of the body are set up for academic use. In the discussion section, research proposals, articles and reports of symposiums can be found. The group is very active in promoting research on the history of Chinese medicine. In addition to holding lectures regularly, the group has organized a number of larger symposiums.

Science and Medicine in Chinese History
http://ccat.sas.upenn.edu/~nsivin/ropp.html
English

This links to a research article written by Nathan Sivin, professor emeritus of Chinese culture and the history of science, at the

University of Pennsylvania. The paper introduces the historical development of Chinese medicine.

Selected, Annotated Bibliography of the History of Chinese Science and Medicine Sources in Western Languages
http://ccat.sas.upenn.edu/~nsivin/nakbib.html
English

This bibliography was created by the renowned scholar, Nathan Sivin, professor emeritus of Chinese culture and the history of science, at the University of Pennsylvania. It is a very detailed bibliography that lists Web sites on science and medicine in traditional and modern China. Although this list, which includes *Compendium of Materia Medica* and *History of Medicine in 20th Century China,* only covers works written in Western languages, anyone who wants to study the history of Chinese technology cannot afford to neglect this comprehensive and useful bibliography. This bibliography is very practical, and its listing is comprehensive. Nathan Sivin frequently updates the content of the bibliography, making this list an essential source for those who study the history of Chinese science. It is also useful for anyone who is interested in the history of Chinese medicine.

Social History of Medicine
Chinese (Simplified)
http://yxshs.zj09.com/index.htm

The site introduces study on the social history of medicine in China. It collects articles, book reviews, news, and syllabi related to this topic.

Somon-Ken (The Study Society of Su wen)
http://www17.ocn.ne.jp/~somon/
Japanese

Huangdi neijing is composed of *Su wen* and *Ling shu.* This academic society specializes in studying *Su wen.* The Web site provides news of the society. It also provides links to other pages introducing different editions of *Su wen* and various explanations on *Su wen* throughout the dynasties. (However, these pages were not found.)

Study Group for the History and Philosophy of Chinese Science and Technology, Technical University Berlin
http://www.tu-berlin.de/fak1/philosophie/china/english/intro .html
English

In 1993, the Technical University of Berlin created a study group that deals with the history and philosophy of Chinese science and technology. This group brings together scholars from all over the world with a common research interest in Chinese civilization. Members of the group collaborate on publications, and there is a two-year program of study for students as well. Current research projects of the group include alchemy and Chinese scientific terminology. This site was created as a resource for students and staff of the Technical University Berlin, Germany. The Web site contains information of course syllabi, list of members in the study group, research projects, and news of conferences. The site also offers excellent guides to organizations of Sinology in Europe, including libraries, study groups and a directory of Web sites on history of science.

Taiwan STS Network
http://sts.nthu.edu.tw/~tsts/
Chinese (traditional)

Taiwan STS network is organized by a group of scholars who are interested in the study of science and technology and its related field. One of the characteristics of the site is that it offers discussion boards organized by different scholars. Under the scheme, there are discussions boards on "Medicine and Social Education" and "Medicine and Healing."

Text and Experience in Classical Chinese Medicine
http://ccat.sas.upenn.edu/~nsivin/epist.html
English

This site is a research article written by Nathan Sivin. The paper introduces Chinese medical texts.

The China Institute for History of Medicine and Medical
Literatures
http://www.cintcm.ac.cn/catcm/ys/enyssjj.htm
Chinese and English

In 1982, the China Institute for History of Medicine and Medical Literatures was created at the China Academy of Traditional Chinese Medicine. Some of the goals of this organization are to study Chinese medical history's development and to bring to light both ancient and modern analyses of medicine in order to further the development of Traditional Chinese Medicine. This institute has a large collection of published material in addition to artifacts with historical value. It is the only institute created solely for Chinese medical history research that exists in China. The Web site mainly introduces the institute, and it divides its introduction into four topics: "introduction," "research," "education" and "academic cooperation and exchanges." The institute publishes the *Chinese Journal of Medical History,* which is the only Chinese journal focusing on history of medicine.

The Golden Elixir
http://venus.unive.it/dsao/pregadio/
English

This Web site is a compendium of references to the history of Chinese alchemy by Fabrizio Pregadio of the Università Ca' Foscari in Venice. The Web site contains information such as a bibliography of Chinese alchemy, a glossary of terms, and reviews of recent literature on the subject of Chinese alchemy. Several Chinese texts are reproduced on this site in Chinese script, such as "Four Hundred Words on the Golden Elixir." This page provides direct access to electronic versions of some classics, including *Zhou yi can tong qie* (Token for the Agreement of the Three in Accordance with the Book of Changes), *Huangdi jiu ding shen dan jing jue juan* (Book of the Divine Elixirs of the Nine Tripods of the Yellow Emperor), *Bao pu zi nei pian* (Inner Chapters of the Book of the Master Who Embraces Spontaneous Nature), *Jin dan si bai zi* (Four Hundred Words on the Golden Elixir), *Huangdi yin fu jing* (Book on Joining with Obscurity), and *Qing jing jing* (Book of Purity and Stillness). In the section of short notes, the life and contribution of Tao Hongjing and Sun Simiao are introduced (two very famous doctors in Chinese history).

Chinese Alchemy and Chinese medicine are interrelated. A major purpose for Daoists to practice alchemy is to acquire longevity. For further information regarding Chinese alchemy, users may refer to the article, "Chinese Alchemy: An Annotated Bibliography of Western-Language Studies" ftp://coombs.anu.edu.au/coombspapers/subj-bibl-clearinghouse/chinese-alchemy-bibl.txt.

Fabrizio Pregadio also has another Web site that describes his academic background and research projects. For those who study medical history, the most essential function of this Web site is to provide electronic versions of Chinese medical classics.

The History of Health
http://www.issp.sinica.edu.tw/hygiene/
Chinese (traditional)

This Web site is dedicated to a research project in Taiwan "The History of Health," by Angela K.C. Leung and many scholars from various disciplines such as history, sociology, and health science. Viewed through the lens of health history, the project aims to study "modernity" through the evolution of health history and concepts of health from the Ming dynasty to the 1950s. The period crosses China in three phrases: traditional, colonial, and post-colonial. The site provides information about this project such as news, conferences, and lectures.

The Institute for the History of Natural Science, Chinese Academy of Sciences
http://www.ihns.ac.cn
Chinese (simplified)

The Institute for the History of Natural Science is the most crucial institute in the field of history of science in China. The institute is a subinstitute of the China Academy for Science, and it has a large number of researchers who are conducting research on different topics in the field of the history of science. The site plays a role in sharing information on the history of Chinese science and medicine. It introduces the history of the institute. It contains publications, researcher information, research projects, and news of the institute. Visitors can access the library catalogs, where they can search *History of Natural Science* and *China Historical Materials of Science and Technology.*

Index